Move
Better

Eat
Smarter

Live
Happier

Strategies for finding balance

Joseph A. Meier

First published by Dog Ear Publishing
4011 Vincennes Rd
Indianapolis, IN 46268
www.dogearpublishing.net

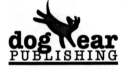

ISBN: 978-1-4575-6001-9

This book is printed on acid-free paper.

Printed in the United States of America

PREFACE

I intend this book to be a basic guide towards a very attainable healthy lifestyle. Do your best to pay close attention to the quotes at the beginning of each strategy (chapter); they're not randomly placed, they're there for your benefit (read them every single day if you so choose). Inside, you won't find in-depth analyses of all the subject matter (physiology, chemistry, or psychology) because, in my opinion, although interesting to me, those subjects can easily go in one ear and out the other, while taking up to 50, 75, even 100 pages of some health books. If this is what you seek, I encourage you to dig deeper on the subjects that interest you the most because we're never too old or too experienced to discover or learn something new or useful. You don't want or need information overload from me; you want to know what you can do *today* to better your health, and that's exactly what you will get. If you want real, reliable and unbiased information, the media (including advertisements, television, many popular health and fitness magazines, etc.) is not where you're going to find it. You're going to find it through *real* research, case studies, and keeping an open mind and experiencing things first-hand.

The strategies in this book are not listed in any order of importance. Each strategy contains its own message that the others do not. Certain people will focus on certain aspects of their health more than others and that is just fine. We are all different. Striving to find an ultimate balance for ourselves – to obtain better health so we can live happily – is really what matters most.

I want to help you discover simple strategies for conquering the aspects of health this book covers. I want to teach you how to exercise smarter, not harder. I want to teach you to conquer eating habits that are holding you back and to share ideas on how to apply my strategies to your own life. I want to teach you how to think through and manage stress so you can minimize stress's negative impact on your life. I want to show you how to keep a positive mindset through the thick and thin in such a negative world. I want to teach you how to stay motivated and on track towards your new and improved lifestyle. Lastly, I want to teach you a little about how lifestyle habits hold people back from reaching their goals and simple strategies for improving your own lifestyle habits each day.

My knowledge comes from a background in Kinesiology and Human Performance. Through my education at the University of Wisconsin-Eau Claire, I learned how the body moves, how it grows, how it recovers from injury and can work to prevent it, and how exercise and diet can work to prevent, reverse and treat an array of diseases and conditions and their underlying causes. My comprehensive education encompassed every subject from human motor development and biomechanics to exercise physiology, psychology and gerontology. I experienced several irreplaceable jobs and volunteer opportunities in college as well as after graduation in which I had a direct impact on the health of those I worked with. My clients include small children, competitive healthy athletes, injured athletes, adults and children with disabilities, older adults, and middle-aged adults with varying health concerns that many more Americans face today.

After graduation, I received my Certified Strength and Conditioning Specialist (CSCS) certification through the National Strength and Conditioning Association (NSCA) in mid-2014 and enjoy applying information I learn from the NSCA's research journals, clinics and conferences to my current practice. I'm a Level 2 Precision Nutrition Certified Nutrition Coach as of October 2017. (The title of the course material is "The Essentials of Sport and Exercise Nutrition" by John Berardi, PhD and Ryan Andrews, MS, MA, RD.) To further my knowledge when it comes to sport performance, I've earned my Level 1 USA Weightlifting (USAW1) certification. Lastly, when it comes to furthering my knowledge in improving athletic performance even more (by looking at muscular and neuromuscular imbalances, muscle weaknesses, and muscle-firing cheat patterns) I've become Level 1 and Level 2 Reflexive Performance Reset (RPR) Certified as well.

I'm constantly trying to learn new information and update my own practices by gaining insight from research, books, journals, articles, and review of the wealth of my own and my clients' personal experiences related to the subject. If I were to rewrite this book in five years from now, I can almost be certain that I would need to adjust multiple portions of it as new information and new research is coming out every month within this field, not to mention what one learns from working in this field changes just as fast, if not faster. If you're ignorant and close-minded, this is not the field for you and it is most certainly not the place to be "set in your own ways", as this keeps you from seeing new truths that are uncovered so frequently.

After years of seeing people struggle with things I found to be fairly simple and easy to apply – and after several years of education, certification, and experience – I started my own coaching business called Lifetime Lean, Coaching for Healthy Living. I wanted to help spread similar information that is found in this book and to coach clients directly. Detailed exercise instruction is also tough to find, and I wanted to make that available, for free, to anyone who visits my site. (https://lifetime-lean.com)

What do I mean by "Lifetime Lean" you ask? First, I mean this is a life-long process. It's a journey that is meant to be enjoyed. It's not meant to be a quick fix or a shortcut to a ripped body. It's meant to make your life a thriving one. Second, by "Lean", I mean to acquire a strong and functional body that makes you happy. Leanness is, of course, fairly subjective, so its meaning will likely be different for everyone. For a lot of people, that means getting "toned". I personally hate that word because the intent behind those who say it is that they just want to lose fat and to see the shapely muscles (they may or *may not* have) underneath that fat without actually building any muscle - which takes a lot of time and patience. To me, being "lean" means that you have a healthy amount of body fat that isn't hurting your health in the long run – it isn't too little or too much. It also means that you have a healthy amount of lean body mass, or more specifically, lean muscle mass that allows you to get what you desire out of life. It also may mean that you have a body that functions the way you want it to and it does everything that is possible within your personal limitations. If you're unhappy for any reason - weaker than you desire, overweight, injured or have the wrong mindset with any of these issues - chances are you're not going to get everything out of life that you may desire.

There is a saying I live by that I knowingly am trying to engrain in the minds of the athletes and clients I work with. "Perfection is impractical; progress is required." Most people who end up upset or disappointed in the progress they make in any endeavor become that way because they have unrealistic expectations. They have an outcome in mind, possibly a timeline for reaching that outcome, and expectations for how easy it should be to get there and what they'll feel like once they do. Nobody is ever going to be perfect. If you ask two different people what their definition of perfection is they will likely disagree. I have yet to hear someone say they think they're perfect in any walk of life. The progress that is required to become better at anything in life is the most important factor in reaching any goal; not just to make progress, but to enjoy the process it takes to get there. If you have an outcome goal of having a "perfect stomach" or just simply to lose 10lbs of fat but you don't enjoy the process it takes to reach that outcome goal (like training your core, doing your cardio, eating mostly whole foods with plenty of protein and vegetables, and drinking plenty of water, etc.), good luck in reaching it *or* maintaining it once you get there. Focus on enjoying the process, *learn* to enjoy the process, become ensconced in the process, and the outcome will become inevitable.

I enjoy taking almost every precaution and proactive measure I can to "improve" or maintain my health through a healthy diet, exercise, getting enough sleep, and reducing stress. I've found it easy to maintain because I have learned to enjoy the process, and I'm hoping you can too once you find your own balance and find enjoyment in conquering personal challenges.

The unfortunate truth about health is that no matter what someone may do, how much they may exercise, or how much of the groceries they buy may be of high quality or organic, health can still take a turn for the worst. We can't control the genes our parents give us or what we may be predisposed to because of our family history, but there are many behaviors that we *can* control to try to improve our quality of life.

"Whether you think you can, or you think you can't—you're right."

-Henry Ford

TABLE OF CONTENTS

INTRODUCTION

In case you're wondering what my goal is for my own personal health before you delve into reading this book, it mainly revolves around maintenance. I'm happy with the amount of body fat I have and have no intentions of cutting down to a very lean 4-6% body fat. I know that's not maintainable or healthy in the *long run* nor is it going to make me a better athlete, triathlete, Tough Mudder, runner, hockey player, tennis player, or recreational cyclist. I'm always working to prevent injuries, get stronger and "shape" myself through resistance training while focusing on maintaining a strong and powerful core.

I train a large number of men and women in the age group of 30-60 years. I know how big they were into sports as kids and I know how their lifestyles shaped the way their bodies function today. I know they neglected stretching more than they should have. Some of them might have drank too much alcohol or eaten too much junk food resulting in unwanted and stubborn body fat they still carry along with poor eating habits or even metabolic diseases. And I know some of them didn't know the first thing about training their "core" muscles (I consider the core from the knees to the shoulders, and all of the muscles that encompass that area), and now they suffer from poor posture, tight hips, recurring acute or chronic injuries, and lower back pain.

I know as a tennis player, I hope to be able to play *decent* tennis until I'm 60+ years old. For that reason, there are certain exercises and training styles I avoid because I know if it doesn't feel great on my shoulders now, it's definitely not going to help my shoulder health in the long run. I will never try to be a solid power lifter or be able to bench 300+ pounds, and I'm completely okay with that. When you know what you want in the future and you know how to enjoy the process (without comparing yourself to everyone around you), you will find success and make progress, as long as you have the patience to make it work for *you*.

The most irritating thing I find with many high-profile exercise and diet magazine articles and media stories is how easy they make "health" sound. I'm not going to tell you that eating a grapefruit every day is going to lower your body fat percentage. I'm not going to tell you the workouts in this book are going to "torch" body fat. I'm not going to tell you that you're going to melt fat and gain slabs of muscle in just 4-8 weeks. All of these claims are just attention getters – and they're misleading and over-exaggerating to everyone who reads them. They fail to mention meaningful information like losing 1-2lbs of weight (ideally body fat, of course) per week or gaining 2lbs of lean muscle tissue in a month is *awesome* progress and has been shown to be far more maintainable than weight loss or weight gain that's more rapid.

Anyone who goes through a lifestyle change that has lasted and impacted them in a way they could never imagine will tell you these claims are misleading too. "Torching body fat" or "increasing your metabolism with one easy step" imply that results will come quickly. Those are the results that usually backfire and send you back to square one, mainly because you became too impatient with the results you were promised. Those are the results I encourage people not to seek. If you want long-term success, strive for the slow and steady results that are just on the borderline between keeping you eager to see where you'll improve next and making you want to question everything you're currently doing. Long-term fat loss and long-term muscle gain are sustainable, healthy and worth it. Losing 5 pounds of body fat per week for 6 weeks before your next vacation is [usually] not.

To better illustrate my point, I'll share with you the story of the tortoise and the hare. When it comes to habit change, the tortoise always wins. The tortoise will get where it needs to be if it's persistent, and it will (as we know) live a long life. The hare, on the other hand, will race as fast as it can to get to where it wants to *end* (the outcome), not taking a second to enjoy the ride (the process) or take in what's happening and learn from it. The hare will only learn, in hindsight, once it reaches the end. The tortoise will learn as it goes and gain invaluable experience along the way.

I want to help you enjoy the process. I want you to be a tortoise, and truly be *okay* with it. If you can become great at little victories that your body responds well to - like drinking enough water or eating enough protein - every single day, you will eventually find success. Once people become impatient with the results that a friend, coach, magazine article or news story promised them if they "follow these three easy steps", everything starts to go downhill.

THE PROBLEM

It's no surprise our nation is having a problem with health: we eat too much, we choose the cheapest and quickest option, disregarding the cumulative effects it will have on our health, and we don't move enough. We spend way too much on health care and drugs to treat the symptoms, but only a sliver on preventing the underlying causes. The nation has started a raging forest fire and is attempting to put it out by throwing ice cubes at it; sure, small portions of the fire at a time might be helped once the cubes melt, albeit temporarily, but the fire will rage on.

I believe a great majority of food and drug companies are interested in money, not health, and they're having the biggest impact on our *obese* problem. The media targets children with the unhealthiest foods to start their eating habits off on the wrong foot at a young age. Schools hardly make an effort to educate kids on what they should and shouldn't eat and why. Schools get a poster with guidelines on it, hang it in the lunchroom, and believe they're doing their best to promote healthy habits to their students. Frozen meals, lack of options and an abundance of junk food with easy availability are what kids are used to these days.

The problem isn't always a lack of willpower from the consumer; it starts with a lack of concern for health from those who are trying to sell a product. Parents have the greatest influence on their children's future health, and frankly, a lot of them aren't doing a very good job. There are a few products that I believe are marketed well but understood terribly by consumers (especially kids).

Flavored sports drinks, various coffee drinks and energy drinks are number one on my list (along with soda, of course) for being a negative influence on the health of our children and country. Sports drink companies portray their products as something that athletes need to drink to stay hydrated and replenish electrolytes and to become better athletes because that's what the pros drink. Electrolytes are lost through being active and sweating, so why do children think drinking a beverage with sometimes as much sugar and artificial flavors and colors as soda is healthy? Because professional athletes drink it – they're the best at their given sports – and it tastes good. Popular sports drinks are key products that get marketed the most, and the most effectively, to consumers – especially to children – who may or may not need them. Of course, nobody knows there are other lesser-known electrolyte drinks and ways to replenish electrolytes besides sports drinks because adding something like sodium, potassium or chloride (to name a few) into your own water isn't advertised even though they would be essentially doing the same thing as drinking a sports drink that claims to replenish electrolytes.

I see athletes year-round and it never ceases to amaze me how many think they need to have a sports drink before or after each practice when they might hardly break a sweat. Sure, they have fast-digesting carbs that may boost energy levels and *possibly* help their athletic performance for a short time, but for a majority of these athletes, water is still going to be the best hydrator, and guess what? You can basically get it for free!

Coffee drinks and energy drinks are also very good at hiding unnecessary sugar, loads of extra calories, varying amounts of caffeine, artificial flavors, and artificial colors. The main pitfall of regularly consuming these drinks is the amount of caffeine and sugar you may unknowingly consume that may eventually contribute to your dependence on such drinks for regular energy. I don't believe having one once in a while is the issue – it mainly becomes an issue when your body can no longer function optimally without such drinks. I'll dive more into liquid calories later.

Breakfast cereal is my number two concern among negative health influences. Most of them contain little fiber, protein or good fats and a majority contain several different kinds of sugar, processed wheat and/or corn, and artificial preservatives, dyes and flavors. They're commonly marketed to children because of the characters on the box and for having "a good source of vitamins and minerals."

Do you know what items are *great* sources of vitamins and minerals that don't need to advertise to get consumers believing they're good for them? Oats and eggs. If you think about it, how many times have you seen a commercial for plain oatmeal you make on the stove or eggs with cooked veggies compared to sugared cereal? Both oats and eggs are a great deal more nutritious than cereal, and they're cheaper too. Plain oats have all the healthy carbs and fiber most cereals do not and none of the added sugar or artificial ingredients. Oats allow you to experiment with flavors and ingredients that you have complete control over. Eggs have all of the protein, fats, vitamins and minerals naturally that cereal does not, and at a fraction of the price. *Shoot, I'd have to take an extra 5-10 minutes to prepare those breakfast foods. Besides, this box has a word find I can do on the back while I mindlessly eat 2-3 servings of it.* Okay, I'm getting off track. You'll learn more about my love for oats and eggs later. Moving onto the third product.

Processed snacks are my number three concern. All the fun-to-eat, colorful, cleverly-packaged, sugar-laden and nutrient-poor snack foods that are so easily available to children are a huge problem. This includes things such as chips, crackers, pretzels, cookies, fruit snacks, granola bars and the approximately 10+ flavor varieties that every company comes out with to intrigue consumers into trying the new flavor. Food scientists are doing a great job of creating tasty, visually appealing and addicting snack foods that kids and adults cannot stop eating.

I'm fortunate enough to have gone through the process of poor health to good health at a young (ish) age to where I probably prevented damage that could have impacted my long-term health for the worse (more than it already had). Looking back at young Joe around age 12-15, a lot of people would say, "Oh, all kids look like that at that age," or "you just hadn't hit your growth spurt yet." This may be true for some children, but with my eating habits at the time, highly unlikely.

After going to college and learning a few things along with reading countless articles, studies, and books on the subject, I'm fairly certain I was on the path to being pre-diabetic or diabetic before I graduated high school. The signs became obvious. Just about every single morning before school I would eat: 1-2 bowls of sugared cereal (9-12g sugar per serving, usually 2-3 servings in a bowl for me), a yogurt (~9-12g sugar), 1-2 pieces of fruit (10-20+g sugar), and a half to a whole cinnamon raisin or blueberry bagel with cream cheese on top (~5-15g sugar). Healthy fats? Nope. Decent amount of protein? Nada. After a high-carb breakfast like that, I was hungry and tired, dosing off in class by 9 or 10 am. The roller coaster ride of insulin spikes and blood sugar drops I was going through every morning would be obvious to me now, but at that age, I just thought I needed more sleep or more food. That damage has already been done, but not without learning from it. There's a reason type II diabetes is no longer just referred to as "adult onset" diabetes - it's because it can wreak havoc on children without them even knowing. The choices they make aren't always their fault – they just need some extra help and they usually aren't getting it.

I've read about plenty of stories (as I'm sure you have too if the subject interests you) of people who had symptoms of diseases such as type II diabetes for years before they finally went to the doctor to learn their blood glucose was in the pre-diabetic or full-blown diabetes range. High blood sugar isn't the only silent symptom associated with this disease either. Problems such as high blood pressure and high total cholesterol, along with low HDL (high-density lipoprotein) and high LDL (low-density lipoprotein) cholesterol, often accompany the disease. And yet, they all can be fairly simply managed if not ignored.

When author Kelly Starrett says, "You can do it temporarily, but it gets expensive," he's usually talking about something related to how the human body functions. In this case, we're not talking about neglecting taking care of your lower back because it's going to put you out of work in 5 years, we're talking about poor eating habits that can lead to disease later on in life. I can't help but laugh when kids say, "Well I'm not fat so it's probably fine" regarding their diet. Yes, I'm sure we all know that one kid with a fast metabolism who won't gain weight no matter what he/she eats. I just hope they realize what they may be setting themselves up for down the road sooner rather than later.

I find it sort of funny how diet and/or exercise can literally be the answer to a *ton* of health issues, yet they're still so hard to commit to for many. What I learned and experienced during my undergraduate career could not be summed up in any health book, article in a magazine, or breaking news story; it was a cumulative learning experience inside and outside the classroom that I have applied in my own life and to my clients that I hope to share with someone new every week.

At risk for osteoporosis? Exercise and a better diet can help. Have a lot of built up stress or suffer from depression? Exercise and a better diet can help. Have a sore lower back? Exercise will help strengthen your core. Want to get stronger to perform everyday tasks with ease? Resistance training will help. Have high blood sugar? Exercise and a better diet will help. Have type II diabetes? Exercise and a better diet will definitely help. Overweight? Exercise and a better diet can help. Over and over again, the answer can be so simple, yet so hard to achieve (1-6, 21, 24, 25).

Ironically, we're essentially paying for our future health. Every poor choice you make when it comes to diet and exercise pushes you closer to poor health. Every good choice you make pushes you closer to optimal health. Both cost a certain amount of money, energy and time. The difference is the money and time spent well will help you stay healthy, avoid injury and have fewer medical bills down the road; the time and money spent on poor choices will add to your waistline, medical bills and health ailments down the road.

Imagine sitting down at a restaurant, paying upfront for the food you want, and instead of getting the food, you get what this food represents for your future health or body composition. You pay for a double-order of hot wings with onion rings and a soda, and the server brings you a mound of jiggling body fat on a silver platter. You order grilled chicken breast on a bed of quinoa and a side of steamed mixed veggies, and the server brings you a slab of lean muscle tissue. You order a double bacon cheeseburger with fries and a melted brownie with ice cream on top, and the server brings you a hardened and nearly closed artery. You're basically buying the fat that goes right onto your love handles (or elsewhere), the lean muscle tissue that will add attractive shape to your frame, or the hardened arteries within your body. This won't happen suddenly or just by eating some "unhealthy" food once in a while, but over time, it will add up. Obviously, this would never happen in a restaurant and is a bit extreme, but I'm just trying to get you thinking.

Most people know exercise and eating well is good for their health, but how many actually know how to do so? I believe I can make this answer as simple for you as you need it to be. Exercise and diet are important, but they are only two parts of the equation to leading a healthier life. I believe there are other aspects of health that are almost as equally important such as stress, outlook, motivation, lifestyle habits, and balance.

Our clocks are ticking, so let's get started.

Exercise

*"Failure is simply an opportunity to begin again,
this time more intelligently."*

-Henry Ford

Where to Begin

First, before beginning any exercise program (especially if you haven't followed one for a while), I urge you to get a regular physical, blood lipid panel (so you know your total cholesterol, HDL and LDL cholesterol and triglycerides) and fasting blood glucose (and/or HbA1c) done so you know a little bit about your current condition. If you've gotten one in the past year but your health may have changed since getting a physical, I still urge you to get an OK from your physician before beginning an exercise program.

The next step I want you to take is to perform a needs analysis for yourself. The purpose of the needs analysis is just what it states – to find out what your *needs* (or wants) are.

For a tennis player, this might focus on aspects of the game such as agility, core power, balance, shoulder stability, and an ability to repeatedly perform powerful movements with the lower and upper body over a long period of time.

For you, this might focus on your hobby of mountain biking on the weekends or kayaking on the river near your home. Feel free to fill out the table below to discover what your needs might include. One side note – just because your workout partner or friend plays the same sport/participates in the same activity as you do does *not* necessarily mean both of your needs are the same – it's still very individualized based upon where you currently stand.

The "Energy System Utilized" refers to the activity being classified as requiring short bursts of power or energy (0-10 seconds), medium bouts of high intensity (30-90 seconds) or long bouts of exercise at moderate to low intensity (>90 seconds at a time). Fill in "short", "medium", or "long" underneath "Energy System Used".

Underneath "Major Movements", fill in the major body movements that are required by the sport or activity. If the activity is playing billiards, the major body movement being looked at would include flexion at the hips along with trying to remain as still as possible while striking the cue ball. This would require static strength of the posterior chain (hamstrings, glutes, and back) as well as flexibility in the posterior chain and flexibility and strength in the shoulders.

> *For every activity you might take part in, core strength and stability (from your knees to your shoulders) should *always* be a factor and a goal of your training program.

Under "Major Skills", focus on writing specific skills that the activity requires. Obviously, for a basketball player, this would include shooting, passing, and dribbling. For a volleyball player, you might include passing, setting, spiking, digging, serving, etc.

Underneath "Common Injuries", write down a few injuries that are common to the sport or activity you spend the most time doing. If you don't know of many, you can always look up common injuries for certain activities and you will find more than you probably wish to see. These are injuries that can either be due to contact with other players, overuse of certain body parts or joints, or acute tissue injuries such as ACL tears in soccer which can occur when a player doesn't even come in contact with any other players.

Underneath "Resistance Training Goal", there are a few things you need to consider when looking at the activity or sport. Does the activity require a great deal of power? Does that powerful movement happen once, or repeatedly without rest? Does the activity require more upper or lower body strength, or the same? Does the activity require a lot of hand-grip strength? Does the activity require very good balance, or is that not important? Does it require many movements in which the body is supported by just one leg at a time? The number of questions you need to ask yourself can go on and on. Take an in-depth look at the activity or sport and each movement required by the individual. From there, you will be able to decide what your main resistance training goals are.

Underneath "Cardiovascular Training Goal", you simply need to look back at what you wrote underneath "Energy System Utilized" and fill in the final box with short, medium or long. If you just wrote "short" (short bursts of energy) in the first box, then you wouldn't need to train for "long" (long-distance running, cycling, etc.).

Needs Analysis

Activity	Energy System Utilized	Major Movement	Major Skills	Common Injuries	Resistance Training Goal	Cardio-vascular Training Goal
Tennis	Short, medium, long	Sprinting, lateral mvmnt, over-head swinging, twisting of the core	Agility, hand-eye coordination, forehand, backhand, serve	Rotator cuff, shin splints, tennis elbow	Upper and lower body power, core power, shoulder stability	Train each energy system
Running	Short, medium, long	Flexion & extension of hip, knee, ankle; sagittal plane movement	Endurance, mental strength, technique	Shin splints, plantar fasciitis, IT band syndrome	Full-body strength, hip strength, core stability	Train the energy system that's specific to your ultimate running goal
Playing with young kids	Short, medium, long	Running/walking, bending at the hips, carrying	Patience, creativity, versatility, ready for unknown, balance	Lower back pain, hip/knee overuse	Well-rounded program, core strength	Train each energy system

Table 1.1

Now, if this looks unnecessary because you just want to learn how to become stronger and you enjoy jogging occasionally, then leave it blank and start with basic resistance training for the whole body 2-3 days per week and include regular stretching and core exercises (more on that later). Not everyone needs to analyze what they're doing, but for some, it can definitely help.

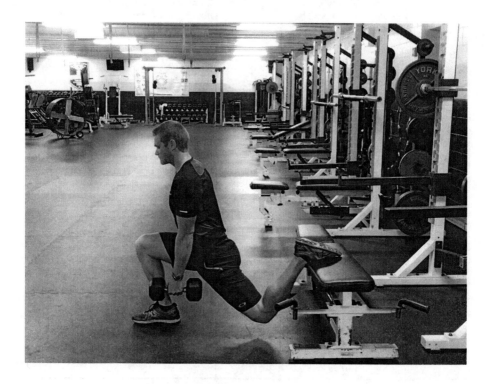

The next step is to decide what exercises you want to include in your training program. After looking at the needs analysis, you should attempt to choose them based on what you've discovered about the activity/sport. For example, a tennis player might include upper and lower body strength exercises, plyometric exercises for the core and the lower and upper body utilizing different types of equipment such as a resistance band and medicine ball, rotator cuff strengthening exercises, and exercises that require balance on one and two legs. The end of this strategy will provide example training programs and styles as well as a resource to use if you're not familiar with how to perform a certain exercise.

What if I left the box blank?

That's great, because your options are endless. I will help you figure out a way to create a schedule and program that works for you later on in the strategy with examples of different types of training (outlined under "A Little On Resistance Training").

One awesome and simple way to gauge *how hard* you should be working and another way to prescribe your own intensity is by using a Rating of Perceive Exertion (RPE) scale – essentially how hard you think you're working. The RPE scale will rate from 1 to 10, with 1 being "this is no work at all" to 10 being "failure/that was extremely hard and I couldn't do any more." I would advise beginners to start anywhere from a 4-6 on the RPE scale for the first 1-3 weeks depending on how active your hobbies and career are.

Another way to think about the RPE scale is by relating that number to the number of reps you left "in the tank", or Reps In Reserve (RIR). For example, if I prescribed someone an intensity of a 7-8 RPE, I would *want* them to stop the set when they feel they could only do 2-3 more reps (10–8 = 2; 10–7 = 3), hence they left 2-3 reps in reserve (1).

How often you should train/exercise is completely dependent upon yourself and your needs. Like I said above, for the average person, training the entire body 2-3 days per week is a great goal. An ironman athlete's training will look insane to most people, where most people might only fit in 30 minutes a day of various exercise, five days a week (which would be fantastic for the average adult, I might add). The other aspects you want to look at are what order you do the exercises you choose, how much weight you lift, how many sets and repetitions you perform, and how long you rest.

The order of exercises you perform each day in your program should, in simple terms, go from powerful (require a lot of force generation) to slow (performed slow and controlled) and complex (multi-joint – like the back squat) to simple (single-joint – like a bicep curl).

This means if you have power cleans, back squat and leg extension in the same workout, power cleans come first (power exercise requiring the most effort and focus on technique), back squat second (a multi-joint strength exercise), and leg extension third (assistance or isolation exercise for the quads).

Performing exercises in this order is how most people, most often, should structure their workouts. It is safest and works to prevent fatigue from occurring on the exercises that require the biggest muscle groups by always performing those types of exercises first. There are other methods such as pre-exhaustion where they are done in the opposite order in which a chest fly (single-joint) would be performed before a bench press (multi-joint) in order to "pre-exhaust" the pec majors. This is an advanced training technique more commonly (and safely) used by those who have years of experience with resistance training. If you're interested in finding out more, I encourage you to dig deeper on your own, or visit https://lifetimelean.com/category/exercise/.

How much you lift is dependent upon your goals. This also goes for the number of sets, reps, and length of rest periods. For most beginners, when it comes to resistance training, a safe place to begin is with one to two sets of each exercise (6-8 exercises covering each major muscle group), 12 repetitions per set (1-2 x 12), performed 2-3 days per week with at least a day of rest in between, with 30-60 seconds of rest in between sets.

If you are *really* deconditioned, and say, haven't lifted anything heavier than a grocery bag in over a year or had just recovered from an injury or illness, you can even start with one set of 12-15 reps (with 4-6 exercises for the whole body) with a very light resistance for each exercise you choose, performed 2 days per week with at least 2 days of rest in between workouts and 45-60 seconds of rest between sets.

Basic Resistance Training Guidelines for Endurance, Hypertrophy, Strength, & Power

Goals	Muscular Endurance	Muscular Hypertrophy	Muscular Strength	Muscular Power (single)	Muscular Power (multiple)
Sets	2-3	3-6	3-6	2-5	2-5
Reps	12-25	6-12	2-6	1-2	3-5
Rest	<30 seconds	30-90 seconds	2-5 minutes	2-5 minutes	2-5 minutes

Table 1.2 (Essentials of Strength Training and Conditioning, 3rd Edition) (25)

Regarding the above table, don't fret if you don't want to lift to get bigger (hypertrophy) and you accidentally did 3 sets of 8 reps last week. Building muscle doesn't work that way, and the likelihood of putting on a bunch of extra muscle by accident is very slim. People spend *years* purposefully lifting heavy or in the "hypertrophy zone" and only manage to put on several pounds of muscle over that time. If you're purposely (or accidentally) eating more calories, you may gain more weight. If you're eating the same amount of calories or less calories, then chances are you're not going to gain an unwanted amount of muscle mass.

To know a little more about how this table works, let's say the first day you barbell bench press 55 lbs 12 times, with the last 2 reps proving quite difficult, but still possible with good technique. You can now say that your 12RM (repetition max) if you could do no more than 12 with good form for the barbell bench press is 55 lbs. Knowing this, if you wanted to resistance train more for muscular endurance, you would want to decrease the weight lifted by 5-10 lbs and increase the number of reps above 12. If you wanted to lift for hypertrophy or muscular strength, you would go in the opposite direction, which would require you to lift heavier loads and perform fewer reps.

I believe everyone should periodize their training program to some extent. Periodizing your program can be very easy, even on your own. Some reasons you should periodize include, but are not limited to, decreased risk of injury, sport performance in/out of season, faster gains in strength and hypertrophy, decreased boredom, and increased mental challenge. A periodized (this example is considered "linear", and each two-week block in this instance is considered a "microcycle") program for someone who has been training for at least 6-12 months might look like this:

Two weeks: 8 exercises, 3 sets of 14, 30 seconds or less of rest between sets, performed 3 days per week

Next two weeks: 8 exercises, 3 sets of 10, 1 minute of rest between sets, 3 days per week

Next two weeks: 6 exercises, 3 sets of 6, 2-3 minutes of rest between sets, 3 days per week

Next week: active rest – play basketball, tennis, or go for a walk or bike ride each day

Next two weeks: 4 sets of 14, 30 seconds rest between sets, 3 days per week

Notice how as the intensity increases, the rest periods also increase. If you're not sure based on your goals how to change up your own sets/reps/rest from week to week, first try sticking with a certain rep and set goal for 3-4 weeks at a time. That's usually enough time for your body to adjust to your routine, experience less soreness, and start to make some noticeable progress.

Then move on to the next set/rep goal for the next 3-4 weeks, and so on, adjusting based on how you *feel*. Exercise selection doesn't need to change at the same time, but it certainly can as long as you're still hitting all major muscle groups 2-3 times per week (if you're a beginner, and/or training your whole body each session).

Remember the guidelines from the table above if you have specific goals in mind and don't know how your body will respond to training yet. If you don't have very specific goals in mind, then periodize similarly to my example above once you have a decent base of training experience so you're training your muscles for strength, hypertrophy, and endurance throughout the year, along with including "active rest" weeks every couple months depending on how you feel.

If you want to get really crazy, you can periodize as much as changing the rep goal each week or workout too (look up "undulating", "block", and "non-linear" periodization to learn more). For example, on Monday you aim for 3 sets of 6 on all lifts, Wednesday you aim for 3 sets of 10, and Friday you aim for 3 sets of 14. The possibilities are endless!

How sore should I be?

This question is posed to clarify when I say "based on how you feel" regarding the adjustments you can make to your periodized training programs.

The answer is simple: *just sore enough*. Just sore enough that you can still perform daily tasks, and just sore enough that you know your training program is challenging you in a way that you haven't been challenged before. If you're constantly sore to the point of being uncomfortable and it affects your daily life, chances are you're overdoing it and you're going to burn out and quit or develop an injury. It might also have to do with your diet and not just your training because certain deficiencies can present themselves as lack of energy, decreased performance while training or increased soreness even when your training program has been consistent over the course of several weeks.

The RPE scale is another great way to manage soreness. If you're training with a goal of an RPE of 5-6, your soreness should be pretty mild. If you're going to an RPE of 8-10 on each set, you can expect to be pretty sore for 1-3 days after your workouts. For the beginner/novice, aiming for an RPE of 8-10 isn't the best idea because it tends to steer people away from resistance training because of the "pain". In this case, the "no pain, no gain" saying doesn't really apply. If you train consistently enough and keep your RPE in check and progress it just as slowly as you do the load you're lifting, you shouldn't be so sore that you don't want to get back into the weight room.

The best thing you can do if you're experiencing out-of-the-norm soreness for weeks at a time is to first dial back the intensity and/or volume of your training (or add in 1-2 extra rest days each week or a more frequent "active rest" week) until your energy comes back, or second (if you don't feel "normal" again after a few weeks of dialed-back training and your diet, sleep schedule, and stress level seem normal), visit a dietician or nutritionist and have him/her analyze your diet. All you may need to do for this is record exactly what you eat and drink for 3+ days (including any supplements or medications) and they'll help you with the rest. One of the most common deficiencies leading to decreased energy and performance (especially in women) is iron deficiency. Deficiencies are usually fairly easy to find and easier to correct with the right kind of help – and not just by guessing on your own. Forgetting about recovery through one's diet is a major progress-killer.

Progressing

After you start, training is pretty easy to adjust. Progressing your own program should be designed to challenge you continuously and keep you from reaching a plateau in forward progress or getting bored.

Something to keep in mind is *how* or *when* to progress. If you perform more than your assigned number of reps (let's say you do 14 on set number 3 instead of the planned 12), then you can start to progress, for example, by adding weight or sets, but choose one or the other. Adding weight and an extra set at the same time each time you think you need to increase the intensity can result in injury. There are a few simple ways you can try to increase the intensity to progress and also help avoid boredom (remember, one at a time!).

Progressing With Repetitions (Reps)

One way to progress would be changing the number of repetitions you perform on each set. This can be done weekly, bi-weekly, monthly, or even daily. If you feel comfortable with the weight you're lifting but don't think the planned 8 reps is challenging you enough, then bump it up to 10 reps per set with the same weight and see how you feel after the workout over the next few sessions.

This is a guess-and-check process with your own body. If you're never feeling slightly tired from expending a lot of energy, sore from providing your muscles with a new stimulus, energized because your body is adapting positively, or stronger from increasing your weights after a workout, then you need to increase the intensity by some means.

Someone else who has been lifting weights for 2 years already who follows a program that consists of 2 weeks with 3 sets of 8 reps, followed by 2 weeks of 3 sets of 6, followed by 2 weeks of 3 sets of 12-15 might yield completely different results than you would. If that works for him or her, that's awesome, but you're a completely different person so discovering how your body handles progressing should be your goal.

Progressing With Sets

Another way you can alter your program is by changing the number of sets. As you've seen in Table 1.2, there are general guidelines you can follow for your goals when it comes to sets/reps/rest. Sets can be changed like reps can, but not as half-heartedly as you might think. For example, for a beginner who has never lifted, during weeks 1 and 2 of lifting, he might decide to do 1 set of each lift. He didn't end up that sore, so during weeks 3 and 4, he might decide to do 3 sets of each. Although this *is* progressing to a higher intensity, adding an extra set or two onto each exercise you're doing that soon can result in getting too sore, too tired, injured, or wanting to quit because it's just plain too hard.

As a general rule, for example, when you're in the middle of a 3-4 week block of performing 2 sets of 10 reps for each exercise, adding 1 set to each exercise and keeping the reps and weight the <u>same</u> for your next 2-3 workouts will allow you some time to see how your body reacts to an extra set of each exercise. Most people will be able to tell a difference in increased soreness after adding just one extra set while keeping reps, weight, and rest the same.

If you can't perform the exact same number of reps on your added set (on set 3 out of 3 you can only perform 8 instead of 10 reps), but you were within a few, then you know the weight you're currently using is challenging enough for your goal of 3 sets of 10 reps, and you may want to keep that same weight until you can perform more than 10 reps on your last set. After a few short weeks or several consistent training sessions, you will likely be able to reach and exceed your goal of 3 x 10 and be able to progress again.

Progressing With Weight (Load)

Progressing your training program with the weight, or load, of each lift should be fairly simple after knowing how to progress with reps and sets. Like I mentioned above, once you start to feel the weight and number of reps/sets you're performing is too easy and you can do more than the assigned reps/sets, it might be time to progress by adding to one factor at a time, such as weight.

As a general rule, increase in small increments of 2.5 to 5lbs on most lifts. Once your technique improves, on large muscle group exercises such as the bench press or back squat, adding 5 to 10lbs as an increment when progressing is much more attainable than adding that same amount of weight to your bicep curl at one time.

Also, when looking at progressing with load, if you're doing it to change from focusing on endurance (12+ reps per set) to hypertrophy (~6-12 reps per set), (as opposed to aiming for the same number of reps while increasing the weight), this will change the number of reps you are doing by *decreasing* them. For example:

You decide after 4 weeks of training with 3 x 10 that you're feeling good and want to continue to work on increasing your strength. For the next 4 weeks, you decide to perform 3 x 6 (which is more so targeting strength according to the guidelines above). Changing your program this way is going to require adding weight to each exercise that you keep the same from the previous 4 weeks because your goal now is 6 reps, not 10. With this lower number of reps and higher load, the intensity will increase and you'll be challenged in a whole new way. If your goal is 6 reps and you don't increase the weight accordingly, you're going to be cheating yourself. I've seen it many times - I progress a client's program to a lower rep range and expect an increase in the amount of weight they're lifting, but they just want to add a small amount of weight (or stay the exact same) they could perform 8-10 reps of, but instead just do the "required" 6 reps and think they're doing it correctly. If it isn't difficult and straining your muscles by rep 5 or 6, then the amount of weight you added for 3 x 6 likely isn't enough to increase your strength over ensuing training sessions.

Remember, with this type of "strength" training goal, your rest would also have to increase to accommodate the new training goal of strength rather than hypertrophy per the guidelines above. When intensity goes up (like going from 3 x 14 to 2 x 6), volume should go down, at least towards the beginning.

It is also safe to say if you're used to doing 4 sets of 15 reps and you decide to train for strength next, it is wise to subtract a set or two from your previous number of sets to see how your body handles the higher loads being lifted. If you were just doing 4 x 15 for three weeks and you decide to change to 8 reps per set, then start your next workout with 2-3 sets of 8 reps. If you feel good after the next couple sessions with the new goal of 2 x 8, then you can move up to 3 x 8 the next week and so on, until you're performing your goal number of sets without unbearable muscle soreness or aching joints.

After you've been resistance training and following a well-rounded periodized program for a while (let's say a year or longer), decreasing the number of sets like in the previous example doesn't need to happen each time you change your training goal – you'll likely be used to changes in intensity by then and will be able to predict how you will feel after progressing.

Progressing With Rest Periods

The last simple way to alter your program is by changing the amount of time you rest between sets. As seen in Table 1.2, there are guidelines for your specific resistance training goal. For example, if you're used to resting 90 seconds between sets of hypertrophy training and you decide to decrease it to 60 seconds of rest, this is going to increase the intensity while staying within those guidelines. The same can be said with endurance – decreasing rest from 30 to 20 seconds between sets will similarly increase the intensity.

One consideration for this is with strength and power. They both require longer rest periods between sets for a couple reasons. First, technique is even more important when performing exercises that are more dangerous like overhead Olympic lifts or lifts when heavier loads are used such as the back squat or deadlift. Second, due to the amount of energy used during lifts that require more muscle to perform, fatigue occurs quicker and recovery takes longer than it does for exercises that don't require as much muscle mass to perform. For these reasons, it would be unwise (especially as a beginner) to decrease the rest below the guidelines between sets of strength or power exercises that require lifting a heavy load or a great deal of focus on technique. As you progress over time, decreasing rest within the guidelines from let's say ~4 minutes between heavy sets to ~3 minutes could be done. The obvious reason you'll know it shouldn't be done is if you decrease rest and your strength suffers on the next set. If this is the case, keep rest during strength/power lifting longer.

Some of you might be thinking, *what about that CrossFit thing? They're jacked and they do those lifts as fast as they can, or they lose!* I'm not going to bash the sport because I like the concept of it – preparing you physically and mentally for the unknown. The only problem I have with this new crowd in the fitness industry is the tendency for the layperson off the street without any weight lifting/Olympic lifting experience to jump in and injure themselves because they either didn't receive proper instruction or they were grouped with experienced lifters and tried to keep up when they shouldn't have.

Those athletes you may see who are repeatedly performing Olympic lifts with heavy loads have been doing it for a long time and they've perfected the form on each lift long before ever doing it as fast as you see on T.V. Before ever performing a strength or power exercise repeatedly with heavy loads, technique must be sound, and you must know your limits and know that comparing yourself to someone who's been doing certain difficult exercises for several years and trying to keep up is a battle your body will likely not win.

On the bright side, CrossFit-type workouts are great for just about anyone because it is basically just a high-intensity form of circuit training. With the correct instruction and supervision, someone at any fitness level can *do* CrossFit; but for some people, some of the known workouts might not be possible due to the Olympic lifts or other exercises they require. If you want to get the same benefit of those types of workouts, refer to the sections below on "Supersets", "Compound Sets" and "Circuit Training".

Progressing With Cardio

When you're trying to become better at whatever it is cardiovascular-wise (swimming, biking, running, etc.), it's important to progress just as you would through resistance training.

When doing low-intensity, steady-state cardio (think an RPE of 1-3 out of 10, with 10 being the hardest possible work) or even moderate-intensity cardio (RPE of 4-6 out of 10), start with a speed and duration that you are 100% certain you can sustain without stopping – if going continuously is your goal. Let's say it's 15 minutes of jogging on a treadmill at 2% grade (because 0% grade on most treadmills is easier than jogging on flat ground) and at a speed of 6.0 mph three days per week.

You could increase the difficulty each week that running goes well and you don't develop any injuries or sicknesses by about 10% of the time you ran. In this case, next week you could run 16.5 minutes and so on while keeping the incline of 2% the same. By increasing the distance you run as opposed to the time, the general rule of a 10% increase per week would stay the same. Be sure if you're just starting up running again (or any activity, for that matter) that you listen to the signals your body gives you and back off when it isn't going well. Some examples of red flags are shin splints, major decreases in energy levels throughout the day or during your workouts, decreased quality of sleep, pain near your Achilles tendon, or a tight IT band that's causing pain near the outside of your knee. The 10% increase per week is a *guideline*, not a steadfast rule.

When you're progressing with something of a higher intensity (RPE of 7-10 out of 10) like High Intensity Interval Training (HIIT), progressing could be done the same as before (by adding maybe a minute of duration per week or two if you're feeling good), or it can be done by changing the work-to-rest ratio (which I would recommend instead of just going for increasing time up to a max of ~30 minutes per HIIT session).

For example, a good way to start off with HIIT if you haven't done it much before is to just perform it one day per week and have a work-to-rest ratio of 1:2 to 1:4. That might look like this: jog at 6.0 mph for 1 minute, then walk at 3.0 mph for 2 minutes, and repeat for 15 total minutes. High intensity interval training shouldn't be done more than 3-4 days per week at any fitness level. The point of HIIT is to push yourself to near or at your max heart rate repeatedly, with periods of recovery in between bouts. Performing HIIT too often can lead to overtraining, injuries, sickness and just plain under-enjoyment of exercise. If you perform HIIT the right way, it can lead to quicker gains in cardiovascular efficiency, increases in speed, and decreases in body fat (2-4).

If you're a beginner, I would recommend starting with HIIT just one day per week and beginning with a session as short as 5 total minutes. See how your body reacts and how much you enjoy the challenge, and adjust from there. If you haven't performed any intense cardiovascular activity in a while, check with your doctor before attempting to train at or near your max heart rate.

A Little on Cardio

<u>What</u>- I believe cardiovascular training should be a part of every single person's training program. Most people have certain goals that will impact what type of cardio they do, so everyone again is going to be different.

I believe in mixing up your form of cardio (also known as cross-training) to avoid boredom and to keep your cardio more interesting and fun. Mixing it up can also help you avoid overuse injuries from doing one type of repetitive movement over and over again until your body bends or breaks, so to say. Some examples of cardio activities you may enjoy include: jogging, sprinting, HIIT, spinning, cycling, mountain biking, swimming, kickboxing, aerobics classes, canoeing, hiking, paddle-boarding, kayaking, Zumba, Tabata training, running to the squat rack before someone else gets there, rowing, the elliptical, stair-stepping, jumping rope, tennis, hockey, pick-up basketball, soccer, and cross-country skiing.

<u>Why</u>- First, cardio can be fun! It can lead you to the outdoors, it can reduce stress, it can lead you to make new friends, and it can help you explore the terrain around you. One reason you *should* do cardio besides the common goal of burning calories or fat loss is because it strengthens your cardiovascular system, and that's something we all should make a priority if we care about our long-term health.

I hate to see people who want to lose weight or be "skinnier" spend countless hours boring themselves to death on the elliptical or treadmill each week (when you should be looking at your diet instead). If you enjoy that type of thing, then keep on keepin' on. If you've never thought, *hmm I should probably jog or bike a few times per week so I have a strong heart when I'm older*, let that be your motivation occasionally to stay on track with your cardio instead of just doing it because you want to lose body fat. Losing fat is great, but having a strong heart and efficient cardiovascular system *could* arguably be more important.

Another reason to do cardio is for weight control (and body composition control). I mentioned earlier, and if you've paid attention to anything fitness-related in the past few years, high-intensity interval training (HIIT) is one of the most efficient ways to improve/maintain your weight/body composition. Cardio can improve many health parameters (and some similar to those of resistance training) that can help you avoid chronic diseases such as osteopenia and osteoporosis, high blood pressure, high cholesterol and Type II Diabetes. Cardio training can improve your health in ways that resistance training cannot, such as increasing the volume of oxygen your lungs can utilize at a given intensity and decreasing your resting heart rate - which in turn will reduce the amount of work your heart has to do at rest.

One side-note on the above paragraph – using cardio as your *only* means to maintain your weight/body composition over time hasn't proven to be the most successful. The human body is smart – and it will become more efficient at using energy to perform movements over time. For example, if you're 25 and you run 3 miles a day, 5 days per week, by the time you're 35 your body is likely going to run that same distance but burn fewer calories doing so. This is one reason why maintaining lean muscle mass via resistance training is a huge part of weight/body composition control as we age. Decreased muscle mass = decreased metabolic rate = less food at mom's Thanksgiving dinner.

One last reason to perform cardio is to maintain/improve immune function (5-7). Moderate intensity aerobic exercise has been shown to improve immune function across various age groups and decrease the length of illnesses when people became sick. However, too much high-intensity aerobic exercise can have the opposite result – decreasing your immune function and leading to a weaker immune response. If you've ever been extremely busy with work, exercise, chores, and/or haven't eaten "well" or lost sleep consistently during busy periods and ended up getting sick, you know what that decreased immune response feels like.

<u>When</u>- When you do cardio is again dependent on your goals and your lifestyle. When it comes to frequency of training sessions, start with a distance/time goal that is *easily* attainable, like 15 minutes of walking

at a brisk pace three days per week. Once that's easy and you feel good enough to go longer, then you can increase the duration, distance, or frequency.

In relation to resistance training, I believe it's in your best interest (most of the time) to do whatever type of cardiovascular warm up you prefer before resistance training, complete your resistance training routine, and then finish with your decided amount of cardio for the day if you're doing both on the same day. The main reason for this is because of the amount of energy and mental focus it takes to resistance train with correct form – especially if you're fairly new to it. If you're exhausted from running three miles and then plan to perform 3 sets of 8 different exercises right afterwards, your form can easily suffer and put you at risk for injury, or worse (not making any strength gains). If you like to run in the morning and lift weights after work and your energy levels are great for both workouts, then that is just fine.

One hot topic – fasted cardio – is becoming more and more common. The premise behind fasted cardio is that performing aerobic activity in the morning after you've fasted for 8-12 hours results in the use of more fat for fuel. The research is still inconclusive in this area (big surprise, I know) but there is some promise to the idea. The best way to find out if fasted cardio helps you improve fat loss is to try it yourself a few days per week (for anywhere between 20-60 minutes) and track your progress over the next few months. If one of your goals is building/maintaining muscle mass, make sure you track *fat loss* progress (using skinfold calipers or another method) while trying fasted cardio. Being in a fasted state can also mobilize amino acids (from proteins) along with fatty acids, so there is a risk of reducing muscle mass over time too.

How- "How" to do cardio is an interesting question to ask. I'm going to explain it very simply: do what you enjoy, for as long as you safely can, while working towards any goals you have, as consistently as you can fit it into your schedule.

Choose a type of cardio that you enjoy (and don't forget to mix it up). Then choose a time that is doable and results in feeling good afterwards and slowly progress with time, type, volume or intensity from there based on your goals. Lastly, choose a frequency each week that fits with your schedule and doesn't make cardio a chore. Once cardio becomes a chore (like in the case of doing too much HIIT, choosing a type of cardio you don't enjoy, running too far right off the bat, or doing it at a time that you hate exercising), your chances of sticking to your routine each week become *very* slim, unlike your future waistline if you fall off the wagon.

If you feel a nagging injury or pain coming on, back off your intensity or frequency, or both, and increase again once that injury has healed or it has been looked at by a healthcare professional and you get the OK to train again. Sometimes too much cardio can result in overuse injuries that appear slowly and gradually, making people believe they aren't serious enough to gain your attention. Not a good idea.

A Little on Resistance Training

Under-Resistance training (a.k.a lifting weights, getting jacked, getting swole) is basically working your muscles against a resistance of some sort. This is why so many different pieces/types of equipment can be used to "resistance train" such as barbells, dumbbells, resistance bands, kettlebells, machines, soup cans, milk jugs, really heavy ice cream cones, your buddy, etc. Everyone can and should resistance train on a regular basis for several reasons.

Why- You don't want to get jacked? That's okay. You can resistance train without having to worry about bulking up. For one thing, if you're a woman, you have significantly less testosterone in your body than a man, so getting huge muscles is VERY difficult to do naturally or as quickly as a man (among other reasons). If you start lifting weights and you become bigger than you want to be, one likely cause isn't the resistance training itself, it's the amount and types of foods you're eating (this is also another reason that every individual needs to see how his/her body responds to a certain set/rep scheme).

To build muscle or gain weight in general, you must be in a caloric surplus. When someone who begins resistance training for the first time has a decent amount of body fat covering their underlying muscles (making muscle definition hard to see), lifting weights may give the illusion that they're actually gaining fat (or just getting bigger – which can be the muscles growing, but this doesn't happen as fast as you'd think).

This reason alone probably steers people away from the weights all the time. They start lifting, their muscles start to grow after a while (which we want!), along with their metabolic rate (which we want!), and they think lifting weights is just making them bigger, not look better. They don't give the process of building and shaping muscle, along with increasing metabolic rate and later on losing fat to reveal their lean muscle, enough time. Patience, people. When you see incredible transformation photos, you don't think those people started lifting and every single one of them just lost fat and gained muscle simultaneously do you?

Of course, resistance training is going to make your muscles stronger, appear more "toned", more resistant to fatigue and more "shapely". If you want to improve the appearance and shape of your body, resistance training must be part of the process. Besides these general and fairly obvious benefits, don't forget it can also reduce the risk of injury, decrease stress, improve joint stability and function, and improve bone strength. It can help improve insulin sensitivity and blood glucose regulation. It can improve your blood cholesterol, including a possible decrease in LDL (bad) cholesterol and an increase in HDL (good) cholesterol. Resistance training leads to a decrease in the chance of disability later in life through increases in bone mineral density, easier performance of activities of daily living (ADLs), improved hand grip strength, improved balance, decreased risk of falls, and a decreased risk of heart disease, certain types of cancer, metabolic disease, and type II diabetes (regular aerobic exercise also contributes to or can more effectively acquire some of these benefits as well) (8-13).

When- Resistance training is a pretty simple thing to plan into your workout schedule. As a general rule (for those who aren't *very* experienced weight lifters or follow a program with a different goal), when lifting a muscle group, let's say chest or upper body, on a certain day, you should allow 48 hours for recovery until your next session focusing on that same muscle group. If you lift total-body Monday, lifting total-body again Tuesday is not the best idea; to let your muscles recover and hopefully not be too sore, you would want to wait till Wednesday or Thursday to do that full-body workout again.

When beginning a resistance training program or new exercises, your soreness can be pretty significant. After adapting to the new type of exercise, your muscles will begin to become less and less sore after each workout and you will be able to adjust the frequency and/or intensity of training sessions accordingly. If you lift weights once, get extremely sore and quit because you didn't like that feeling, you simply need to start at a lighter intensity and give your body more time to adapt to the new activity (recall the RPE goal for beginners from earlier and again listed below).

As I also mentioned earlier, resistance training *before* any fatiguing cardio is performed is usually the safest choice, especially if you haven't perfected your technique yet. Jumping into a lifting session when you're tired from HIIT (or any other possible choice) can result in injury.

<u>How</u>- How to lift weights is a very broad category. Knowing the correct form, or technique, of an exercise is important for targeting the correct muscle groups and avoiding injury. Always remember, **form** comes before **weight**. You may think you can lift a lot of weight on a certain lift because you threw hay bales as a kid, but if your form isn't correct before you increase weight, you increase the risk of injury. If you aren't sure if your form is correct, meet with a qualified fitness professional, or visit https://lifetimelean.com/learn/instruction/ for exercise instruction.

Intensity should be a focus of your attention while resistance training to ensure you're doing it safely, so you don't develop chronic/acute injuries, and so your soreness is manageable.

For beginners, aim for an RPE of 4-6 out of 10 for the first few weeks of your exercise program. Once your soreness becomes less significant, you can move upwards in small increments on the RPE scale approximately 1-3 weeks at a time. Once you become more experienced and know how your body will react to certain intensities and loads, it becomes easier to understand the RPE scale and you can use it within your own programming to determine how hard you should work.

If you were accustomed to weight lifting for several months and were getting ready to work on building muscle and increasing strength for the next 13 weeks, programming your own intensity (periodizing intensity based on RPE to keep soreness in check) instead of just using sets/reps may look like this (along with *expected* soreness):

Weeks 1-2: 3x12, RPE of 4-5 (easy lifting, focus on technique; very light soreness, if any)

Weeks 3-4: 3x10, RPE of 5-6 (add small amount of weight; mild soreness)

Week 5: 3x10, RPE of 6-7 (add small amount of weight; same mild soreness)

Week 6: 3x8, RPE of 6-7 (add small amount of weight; mild soreness)

Week 7: 3x8, RPE of 7-8 (add small amount of weight; moderate soreness)

Week 8: 3x6, RPE of 7-8 (add small amount of weight; moderate soreness)

Week 9: 2x12, RPE of 5-6 (easy lifting, focus on technique; no soreness)

Week 10-11: 3x6, RPE of 7-8 (replicate Week 8 loads on Week 10, adjust for Week 11 based on soreness, and then adjust again for Weeks 12-13; mild soreness)

Week 12-13: 3x6, RPE of 8-9 (add small amount of weight; moderate soreness)

*Week 14: 3 sets of eating ice cream, RPE of 10 (make gains; no soreness – just happiness)

Week 9 in the above example may seem out of place, but it's a very necessary piece of the periodization puzzle. It's essentially an "easy" week with the purpose of giving your mind and your body a break before continuing again and increasing intensity. If you've been training consistently but seem to be getting bored, end up in a plateau, or feel an injury coming on, take a week off (like Week 9, or just completely off from lifting) and you should come back far more prepared for the increase in intensity. *Week 14 is a joke, unless you love ice cream as much as I do.

For another simple example, if you're aiming for an RPE of 7-8 and doing a set of 10, reps 8, 9, and 10 should be quite tiresome and maybe even cause some burning in your muscles or shaky arms or legs, but not so hard that your form starts to go to crap or you fail and drop the weight. Lifting to failure on every set *is not* necessary, nor is it enjoyable for most people. If you finish a set and think to yourself, *okay, I feel like I'm at about an 8/10, I may have been able to squeeze out 2 more reps,* and your form was still solid, then you're right where you need to be.

Something worth mentioning during weight lifting is breathing. When holding your breath during the hard part of a lift (generally going from eccentric to concentric; for a squat, lowering your body would be eccentric because muscles are lengthening, and standing back up would be concentric because muscles are shortening), a "fluid ball" in your torso is formed to help support your spine. When holding your breath through the "sticking point" (going from the eccentric part to the concentric part of the movement) your blood pressure can increase immensely. For that reason, it is advised that breathing out *through* the sticking point and during the concentric part of the lift is the safest way to lift, especially for beginners.

An example during the back squat would look like this: you brace your core, get the bar on your back, step back, and drop down into the squat. Once you reach the bottom of the squat, you push upwards and start to exhale slowly on the way up as you keep a braced core throughout. You take another breath once you're standing upright and then drop down for your next rep.

Experienced lifters do purposely not breathe through the sticking point to keep their torso more rigid (and to increase spinal support), but most often they are experienced enough to know the benefits and the risks of holding their breath through the sticking point and concentric movement and sometimes feeling light-headed, seeing stars, or passing out can be a result. Chances are you're not performing a 1RM without proper instruction and supervision, so stick to breathing out through the sticking point and during the concentric portion of your lifts.

I'm going to explain a few different ways to resistance train and some of their benefits (which will be laid out later on in the strategy) besides just the general format of doing 2 x 12 of one exercise while resting for a certain period between sets, and then moving onto the next exercise after completing all sets.

1. Circuit Training – You have a set number of exercises (let's say 8) and/or reps (let's say 12) that you perform one after the other with minimal (<30 seconds) rest in between exercises. After you go through all 8 exercises, you can rest 1-3 minutes before going through again. Start off with 2 rounds and adjust from there.
   a. Some benefits of this type of training are improved muscular endurance, time-efficiency, decreased likelihood of "getting too big", and it keeps your heart rate high during the entire workout from having minimal rest, therefore possibly increasing the metabolic impact on your body and, in a way, counting as "cardio" for those cardio-haters out there.

2. <u>Supersets</u> – You choose two exercises that work opposing muscle groups (chest and back, biceps and triceps, or an upper and lower body exercise) and perform them back-to-back with no rest in between.

    a. The benefit of this type of training is similar to circuit training, where you can perform X amount of sets in less time because while you work one muscle group, the opposing muscle group gets to rest.

3. <u>Compound Sets</u> – You "compound" two different exercises that work the same muscle group together, with minimal rest in between exercises.

    a. This is quite a bit more tiring than alternating opposing muscle groups like with supersets. You will notice your muscles will fatigue more quickly and you will experience a bigger "muscle pump" as well. I would also advise decreasing the load lifted by 10-30% (at least on the second exercise of the set) when doing compound sets if you don't have someone watching your form or a spotter for the lifts that require one.

4. <u>Pre-Exhaustion</u> – You "pre-exhaust" a specific muscle, usually with an assistance exercise, before performing a more complex exercise that works the same muscle group. An example would be the pec fly before the bench press or performing a lateral shoulder raise before the barbell shoulder press.

    a. This type of training can be very high intensity, and can result in more micro-tears in the muscle fibers resulting in increased soreness and increased muscle hypertrophy and strength. It is a widely-used method among bodybuilders and those who are just trying to increase their strength or muscle mass.

5. <u>Power Training</u> – You attempt to move a weight *quickly*. When training for power, it is important that you start with a lighter weight than you might usually lift for a given exercise (maybe 40-50% of your 1RM or predicted 1RM). While training for power, it is also important to reduce the number of reps you perform per set due to the great amount of energy it takes to move a weight quickly *and* with correct form (if form isn't correct throughout – which is likely to happen if you do too many reps in a set and attempt to do them quickly – you

greatly increase the risk of injury). The number of reps *and* weight should be lower than what you might do to train for strength or hypertrophy.

a. The benefit of training for power is universal. Many activities we perform every day require power without us even thinking about it. For example, walking up stairs, starting a lawn mower, jumping, throwing, catching your balance after tripping, and playing almost any sport or activity that involves quick movement and quick reactions such as softball, volleyball, basketball, tennis or golf.

*One other note regarding improving power – increasing strength (with use of heavy loads and long rest periods) *does* contribute to the muscle being able to produce power as well. The above example is just referring to moving weights quickly (focused on a quick and explosive concentric portion of the lift), not moving very heavy loads slowly.

Time Management

Your own personal workout schedule should fit your lifestyle so it doesn't always feel like a hassle. You might be thinking already, jeez this looks like it's going to take a lot of time to get through that many exercises, and then I have to do cardio for 45 minutes? Fortunately, no. It's quite simple: decide whether you can get your workout done in the morning, at lunchtime, or after work. After you decide when you prefer to exercise, then you can plan how much time is spent doing which activities.

Once you decide what your goals are and how much time you want to spend lifting weights, doing cardio, etc., then you can decide how many days per week you're going to resistance train. For example, if you can only lift weights two or three days per week, it would be wise to train your entire body each of those days, making sure there are at least 2 days in between workouts. You could train Monday/Thursday, Tuesday/Friday, Monday/Wednesday/Saturday; the best route to take is whatever works with your schedule and whatever you can stick with in the long run.

If you want to commit to lifting four days per week, then you can separate your lifting even more to upper and lower body days. For example, upper body on Mondays and Thursdays, and lower body Tuesdays and Fridays. This is possible because the muscle groups being lifted on back-to-back days won't overlap drastically so fatigue shouldn't hinder your next-day workout.

For the more dedicated weight lifter who wants to train 5-6 days per week, you can even consider separating the resistance training days by body parts such as chest one day, legs the next, shoulders the next, back the next, and arms (and legs again) last. Generally, I wouldn't recommend training that way as it takes a lot of time and most people want efficiency out of their program – unless you're much more into lifting weights than doing cardio for consistent daily exercise – then by all means lift some weights 5 days per week and split it up accordingly.

The thing most people don't realize is that you *can* get lifting done in 20 minutes and move on with your day (this is where circuit training and supersets come in handy). Think about how much time each day you spend doing things like waiting in lines, using the restroom, cooking, watching TV, or surfing the internet. Twenty minutes of quality lifting is all you need with a busy schedule, and it doesn't even have to be every day. Refer to the section under "Resistance Training" to help you out with shortening your workouts and making them burn your muscles and cardiovascular system at the same time.

The key to sticking with a program is adjusting it to fit your lifestyle so you're likely to continue it long-term. No matter how "awesome" your program is, it's ultimately going to be ineffective if there are too many barriers preventing you from staying consistent.

Your Training Schedule

Day	Monday	Tuesday	Wednesday	Thursday	Friday	Saturday	Sunday
Weights							
Cardio							
Other							

Table 1.3

In table 1.3, fill in the days of the week you believe, with your schedule, you can resistance train, perform cardio, or "other" which could include any random activities, sports, or fitness classes you like to attend. If you don't know where to start, aim for a minimum of two days per week (on non-consecutive days) of resistance training for the entire body and between 3-5 days per week that include some type of cardio (cardio here could be biking to work, 3 separate periods of walking for 10 minutes at a brisk pace throughout the day, or a planned 4-mile run).

For example, your chart might look like this: next to "Weights", you could fill in "full body" on Monday and Thursday. Next to "Cardio", you could fill in "run 2 miles" on Monday, "bike to work" on Tuesday, and "swim 20 laps" Thursday and Saturday. And next to "Other", you could fill in "1-hour tennis" on Sunday.

I encourage you to photocopy this chart or create your own and use it each week/month for your own program, at least in the beginning, if you have trouble "remembering" (yeah, right) to exercise until you make it a habit (remember, reducing the number of barriers is a goal here). Hang it near your desk or on your fridge at home to keep yourself accountable and on track with your goals. If one week or month is busier than the next, fill in the chart again with a program that will work with your schedule.

When planning your week, just look back and make sure there are at least 2 days of resistance training and at least 3 days that include some type of cardio (remember, there are multiple ways to get "cardio" in – it doesn't just have to be running or biking). The better you plan, the better your chances of sticking to your program and avoiding the classic, "Oops... I must've gotten busy" while checking out your new muffin top 4 weeks after attempting to start.

If you're an avid gym-goer who attends group fitness classes, you're likely going to get a mix of both cardio and resistance training depending on the types of classes you go to. I believe those types of classes can be beneficial, but I also believe everyone should still take some time to resistance train outside of group fitness in a controlled environment where they know they're progressing in weight and building strength doing specific movements. Group fitness classes are great for full-body exercise, but when it comes to progressively building strength and tracking progress, resistance training in the weight room with free weights or machines is tough to beat.

Tracking Progress

Progressing in your training program and your health is usually fairly easy to feel and see after you get into the swing of things. If you're the type who needs something written down in front of you that you can physically carry with you or read to know how you're doing, then writing down your progress might be necessary. If you're not the type of person who wants to carry around a notebook or sheet of paper everywhere in the gym with you, that's okay, because I'm definitely not that type of person either.

"Tracking" can just be a check in with yourself every week, month, or several months and a reflection on your goals and where you wanted to be after starting a week, month, or several months ago. It could be measuring yourself with a girth measuring tape or weighing yourself on the scale. It could be performance based (my #1 choice), which could be remembering or writing down at home how much weight you squatted in September, and comparing it to what you can do now in December. Whatever works for you is what you should stick with. The more specific your goals, the more vital it is going to be to keep track of your progress on a daily, weekly, and/or monthly basis.

Why you should ditch the scale

If your goal is to lose fat, I urge you not to rely solely on the scale as a means to track progress. Get your body fat percentage checked with a BIA, DEXA or skinfold caliper to get an idea of where you're at. If you're eating too much while lifting weights and gaining weight *isn't* your goal, you might gain more weight than you want initially – even if that includes lean muscle mass, leading you to believe lifting weights is making you go backwards.

As you increase your lean mass, your resting metabolic rate (RMR) is going to increase as well. So, when trying to lose weight, you may be losing fat and gaining lean mass at the same time (not *literally* the same time – that's not possible, but within the same period of, let's say, 6 months), making your daily weigh-in fairly useless. Save yourself the stress and go by how you feel, how you look, how your clothes fit or your measured body fat percentage by one (or another) of the means listed above.

The scale doesn't measure fat loss; it measures *weight* loss. The other, possibly more important, measures of success not already mentioned that the scale doesn't tell you include how your current/old clothes fit, how much fat mass you've lost, how much muscle you've gained, how much your blood pressure or cholesterol have improved, how much more efficient your cardiovascular system is (easily noticeable by a decrease in your resting heart rate), how much stronger you've gotten, how your joint stability has improved, how your balance has improved, how the strength of your bones, ligaments and tendons have increased, how flexible you are or how much more resistant to injury you are.

If you forgot about the scale and focused on these types of improvements as your main goal instead of weight loss, with a healthy diet, the weight will come off and the muscle will come on. The processes you must follow to acquire some of these benefits are the processes that will lead to a leaner body.

If you're also one of those people who always just want to "tone" their body everywhere, consider deleting that word from your vocabulary to save yourself a bit of frustration.

The act of "toning" is essentially an increase in lean mass and decrease in fat mass (although, most people using that word are simply interested in losing fat, even if they don't possess the underling muscle they want to reveal yet).

If you want nice looking triceps or a defined back, go into the process with the mindset of wanting to get stronger and eat healthier. Focus on getting really good at finding a consistent weight lifting and cardio schedule and planning a healthier diet.

Losing weight doesn't guarantee you a "toned" looking body. By lifting weights, you might even *gain* weight and end up looking more toned than you did before. If you want to be toned, what you really want is to be *leaner*, and being *leaner* means your goal should be to increase your *lean* mass and decrease your *fat* mass. Once again, the scale isn't going to be your best tool for tracking this progress. (Of course, if you've got 75-100+lbs of body fat to lose, the scale will be a good means to measure progress in the beginning, but still shouldn't be the only means to measure progress as you become leaner.)

Something that can be used to track progress which is pretty well known in the industry (the letter definitions change from source to source) is a SMART goal. I encourage you to try it and create your own SMART goal and fill it in below.

<u>S</u>pecific: "I want to get into shape" is not specific. "I want to lose 15 lbs in 3 months" is.

Your specific goal:

<u>M</u>easurable: You can track your goal by measuring it somehow. This could be a 1RM strength test, girth measurements, or weighing yourself on the scale. "Weighing myself every Sunday morning" at the same time to see if you're on track is progress that is measurable.

Days/times you will remember to measure:

Type of progress that can be measured:

<u>A</u>ttainable: Your goal is within reach for <u>you</u>.

On a scale of 1-10 (1=I can't do this, 10=I can definitely succeed), how would you judge your confidence in reaching the goal you've described above?

1   2   3   4   5   6   7   8   9   10

*If you're below a 9, you should re-think your goal so you're between 9-10 on the scale.

<u>R</u>ealistic: Your goal isn't completely unreachable like, "I want to increase my max squat 100 lbs by next week."

What are you going to accomplish in the timeframe you've chosen, and what makes you believe you can succeed?

Timely: The time you choose to allow yourself to reach your goal isn't too short or too long. Keep in mind: a safe weight loss goal per week is 1-2 pounds (unless you have 100+ extra pounds to lose, in which case that number will be higher towards the beginning). This gradual weight loss will increase the chances of you keeping the weight off once you reach your goal. If you have a wedding in three months you want to slim down for, then a safe weight loss goal might be about 1-2lbs per week, or 12-24lbs by the end of the three months.

Where will you be/how far along towards your goal do you want to be on:

Week 1:

Week 2:

Week 3:

Week 4/1 month:

Week 5:

Week 6:

Week 7:

Week 8/2 months:

3 Months:

4 Months:

5 Months:

6 Months:

1 Year:

2 Years:

Safety

Safety should always be the number one priority. The correct technique for each exercise is important for avoiding injury and making sure you're working the targeted muscle/muscle group. When looking for a qualified fitness professional to meet with, look for someone who is a Certified Personal Trainer (CPT), Certified Strength and Conditioning Specialist (CSCS), or someone who has an educational background in the exercise science or kinesiology field. If you're unsure of the certification someone might have, do your own research online or ask someone you trust in the field so you can make your own educated decision and whether or not you want to trust that individual.

Know that when you begin a training program or come back after a long hiatus, your muscle soreness will likely be significant. The more consistent you are with your new training program (as long as you don't overdo it), the less you'll be sore after each ensuing workout. It may take you a month, or it may take you four months until you're noticeably less sore after training. If you're progressing correctly and aiming for the right RPE during each set, you should be past the initial soreness stage after about 8-16 training sessions.

Being sore isn't the only indicator of progress or success either. A little soreness to remind yourself that what you did yesterday is working is great, but if you're constantly sore and lacking energy to train, your chances of sticking to your current routine are going to plummet, and you need to back off the frequency, intensity, or both. Not paying attention to soreness or how you feel on a regular basis on a certain program can easily result in overuse injuries.

Age is a big topic when it comes to resistance training. Believe it or not, older adults (>65 years old) *can* safely resistance train just like anyone else can with the proper instruction. Of course, there are things to keep in mind with older adults you don't usually need to keep a close eye on with younger adults or athletes, such as medications they may be taking, their bone and joint health, or prior injuries or health concerns that might impact their ability to perform certain exercises or exercise at a certain intensity.

Resistance training should be done by older adults *especially* for the sake of improving or maintaining the strength of muscles, bones, joints, and connective tissue, along with improving balance and the ease of their activities of daily living. Older adults can safely perform a lot of the same type of training outlined in this strategy as long as they're comfortable with it and have proper instruction.

The weights, sets, reps, and rest should all be started on the easier side when compared to younger adults or athletes. This would mean less weight, fewer sets, higher reps, lower RPE's, and longer rest periods during training sessions and between sessions than the recommendations stated in this strategy. Keeping this in mind, the program of an older adult should still progress in some way to keep them improving. Just because someone is 70 years old, does not mean they can't progress to lifting down to a 6RM or lower over time. Again, safety first.

On the other hand, how young is it safe to start resistance training? There is no conclusive research whether resistance training too early can inhibit growth or increase risk of injury. Although, there is evidence that after a child has gone through/is going through puberty (fast growth spurts, reaching Peak Height Velocity (PHV), increasing muscle/bone mass, increasing hormone levels, eating a ton, etc.), it's okay to start learning the correct and safe way to resistance train without undue risk (14-16).

The extent of their training at this point should focus on being able to control their body weight (with squats, jump squats, push-ups, planks, lunges, etc. with correct form) and learning correct technique for large muscle group lifts such as bench press, deadlifting, and lat pulldown. Having a solid base of knowledge, coordination, and injury-resistant tissues and joints is most important for a growing child.

There's no need to have them on a periodized program and testing their 1RM every three months at this age. The focus should be on learning and enjoyment, not getting as strong as possible so they can make the varsity hockey team before they're a freshman in high school.

This is also usually the time kids begin to be "athletic" when they might have been a fumbling buffoon just a year before with less hand-eye coordination than a common house cat. Before kids get to that state, just focusing on their sport-specific movements and activities to keep them active and enjoying sports and an active lifestyle is all they should need to worry about. Being active at a young age is vital for the improvement of hand-eye coordination, brain development, social development and muscle, connective tissue and bone development.

It has also been shown that early sport specialization *doesn't* increase the chances of future success in that sport but *does* increase the risk of burnout and overuse injuries (17, 18). As parents and coaches, it's best to keep kids active, having fun, and encourage participation in multiple sports.

Recovery

I mentioned recovery when it comes to training frequency, rest periods between sets, and when you need to back off training to avoid overtraining and injury, but there's another subject when it comes to recovery regarding weight training and exercise. It has to do with the extra work one does to keep joints and tissues feeling good.

Foam Rolling (Self-Myofascial Release)

If you don't spend a few minutes paying attention to the flexibility of your muscles and the range of motion of your joints each day, you may be missing out on healthy long-term maintenance. Foam rolling is not only a very inexpensive form of tissue massage, it has been shown to increase blood flow, increase flexibility (range of motion) without decreasing power output pre-exercise, and *possibly* decrease muscle soreness post-exercise (but I wouldn't count on it) (19-24). The research on foam rolling and foam rolling techniques is not yet conclusive and more work needs to be done to determine the mechanisms behind its impact on tissues.

Foam rolling can be done pre- and/or post-workout for the reasons stated above. Give it a shot before and/or after a few workouts and see how it makes you feel. The biggest difference I've noticed personally after regularly using a foam roller is increased range of motion, decreased soreness/tightness in certain areas and the prevention of shin splints.

Warning: foam rolling, if you haven't done it before, can be quite painful and uncomfortable, especially on areas such as the side of the thigh (IT band/TFL). Start foam rolling with an "open celled" roller (which are much softer and have a lot of give) until you can no longer feel the deep massage you're after, and then progress to a firmer roller until you can roll on a (usually black) hard or "close celled" roller. Don't worry, the more often you roll tight areas, the less it hurts and the better you feel during and after rolling. You can't expect tight, neglected muscles and tissues to feel "good" in the beginning as you attempt to loosen them, but stick with it.

When foam rolling, simply start at the bottom of your calves right next to your heels and slowly work your way up to the top of your back.

Stay on each area (lower calves, upper calves, lower hamstrings, mid-hamstrings, upper hamstrings, left/right glute, lower back, mid-back, upper-back, lats) for about 45-60 seconds rolling slowly up and down, and when you find an especially tight or tender spot, pause on it for a few seconds, and then continue on. As you start to move upwards, tilt to each side of your legs and back as well to cover as much of the muscle as possible. Upon reaching your back, cross your arms (give yourself a big hug, you deserve it) so your shoulder blades spread apart and you can more easily reach the muscles of your middle-back. After you get through the backside of your body, which should take ~5 minutes, flip over onto your front.

For the front of your body, start in a plank position on your elbows, with the roller right above your knees. Before this area, you can roll the front and sides of your lower legs but it's a lot more difficult than using a rolling pin or hand-held roller for that small area, which I prefer simply for ease of rolling. With the roller starting right above your knees, just roll forward and back in your plank position about 6 inches at a time. Then spread your legs apart a bit and tilt your body so you can reach the inner quad muscle, and again repeating by tilting the other direction to focus on the outer quad muscle. Move slowly upwards just as you did for the backside of your body, taking 45-60 seconds per area and pausing on extra tight areas. Continue this all the way up to the front of your hips, which can be an especially tender area.

For the last part of your legs, you will assume a side plank position on your hands or elbows with the leg that is closer to the ground straight and resting on the roller just above the knee, and the top leg with your foot planted on the ground in front of your lower leg and below the foam roller. Your top leg is just used to decrease the pressure on the lower leg until you get used to it, then you can just stack both of your legs and keep them straight while you roll the sides of your legs (quads/hamstrings), all the way up to the top of your hip. This IT band/TFL/glute medius area gets especially tight on those who spend a lot of time sitting, running or biking without taking time to stretch. Neglecting this area can cause lateral knee pain that's extremely annoying, and all it takes to prevent could be a little foam rolling and stretching – mainly of the area near the side of your hip and your glutes.

Instrument Assisted Fascial/Soft Tissue Mobilization (IAFM/IASTM)

Another form of myofascial release that's used more often in a clinical setting is by use of stainless steel tools like the Myofascial Releaser and Graston Technique tools. This method of myofascial release could be described as a "more intense" method than what's sought after through foam rolling or manual massage. This technique can be done in small areas and to help relieve chronic and acute pain such as with plantar fasciitis, tendinitis, and tennis elbow.

Static Stretching

Static stretching also holds some importance in recovering from workouts – but it might not be what you think. If you want to increase your flexibility, you've got to stretch pretty much every single day to achieve and maintain a certain high level of flexibility. Hold each static stretch at a point of just mild discomfort for 30-60 seconds, and repeat 2-3 times per muscle group.

Static stretching before or after a workout isn't going to prevent you from being sore, but it will help prevent you from becoming a full-body piece of tightened lean mass that has very limited range of motion and poor dynamic flexibility. An example would be being unable to reach behind your head with your right hand to touch the top of your left shoulder. Those would be some extremely tight and inflexible shoulders and lats. There are also two other ways I prefer to stretch out the shoulders to keep them as limber and pain-free as possible (especially for an overhead athlete).

*One other reason to lift weights, especially free weights like dumbbells, is the ability to perform exercises through a greater range of motion, in turn improving the flexibility of a joint and surrounding tissues.

Unconventional Stretching

The first way requires a resistance band and some type of immovable pole, door or piece of gym equipment (the anchor). Grab a resistance band with one hand, anchor it on something shoulder height or above and step back while facing the anchor. Keep your knees and hips square to the anchor and relax the arm and shoulder that is holding the taut resistance band until you feel a very nice, slight pull on your shoulder (it *shouldn't* feel like your humorous is popping out of the socket).

Retract your shoulder blade (bring your shoulder back so now knees, hips and shoulders are all aligned and square to the anchor and your shoulder blade is "tucked" in toward your spine), hold it for a moment, and relax it again. Repeat this 6-10 times. Then for the rest of the stretch, while holding the resistance band in the same hand, you will just rotate your body in each direction and hold the stretch for 20-30 seconds. You should end up facing down towards the ground, completely left, right and away from the anchor. This stretch is a great upgrade from the usually-seen standing deltoid stretch in which you straighten your left arm out in front of you, reach across and grab your left elbow with your right hand, and pull your left elbow towards your right shoulder. I would recommend trying *lightly* performing this resistance band stretch for about 10-15 seconds in each range of motion before working out, or at length as described above for 20-30 seconds in each ROM post-workout.

The second way requires a dumbbell or kettlebell. Start with approximately 10lbs the first time you do this until you feel comfortable and your shoulders become a bit more stable. Set your feet far beyond shoulder width apart and place the weight in between your legs. Flex at the hips, keep a neutral spine, and grab the weight while keeping your opposite hand on your knee for extra support.

Now, you're just going to slowly swing the weight around in a circle with your shoulder relaxed, or protracted, just like you would at the beginning of the resistance band stretch described above. After 6-10 circles one direction, change directions and repeat on both sides (careful not to hit your shins or knees). Again, make sure you keep a neutral spine throughout so you don't get a sore back swinging around a 25 lb kettlebell later on. Then, repeat the same process with your shoulder pulled back (retracted). I would recommend doing this before and/or after a workout, but only after you get the feel for it and find a weight that noticeably makes a difference in your shoulder flexibility and stability.

To learn more about taking care of your body when it comes to mobility and avoiding chronic injuries, see *Becoming a Supple Leopard*, by Dr. Kelly Starrett with Glen Cordoza and *Deskbound*, by Dr. Kelly Starrett with Juliet Starrett and Glen Cordoza.

Should I train when I'm sore?

There are three things you should try doing that can benefit you when you want to exercise but you're still too sore to "feel like it" from your last workout.

First, you can foam roll as described above. If you find foam rolling relaxing or notice an increase in ROM or decrease in tight/sore muscles, then more power to you.

Second, you can train the muscle groups you were planning on training *very lightly*. The problem with this, of course, is you are, in a way, just going through the motions without pushing yourself, in which case you might as well wait until tomorrow and put in the work then. If you're dying to lift or you're about to go on vacation and you'll miss the gym, light lifting on sore muscles isn't going to hinder your future progress or likely result in injury. Just remember to lift *very lightly* (I'm talking using a weight you would normally lift 8-10 times and cutting that weight in half for each exercise) so you don't risk poor form that results in injury.

Lastly, you can partake in some light- to moderate-intensity cardio (below a 6 on the 1-10 RPE scale). Just like foam rolling can help loosen the muscle and increase blood flow, light cardio (not HIIT) will also help loosen tight muscles by increasing the blood flow to the muscle and surrounding tissues and in turn increase nutrient delivery for recovery. Then, you can hop on the foam roller and/or static stretch afterwards to cool down and continue to loosen up.

The majority of recovery boils down to what you're eating when you're not training. We'll get into that later, but now you have a few strategies to "damage" your muscles and then assist their recovery.

Bill was the unfortunate result of driving on a life-long road of poor health choices. His 75+ pounds of excess weight was mainly held around his mid-section – known as visceral fat. This is the fat that surrounds the organs and increases the chances of developing a vast array of diseases. The way his excess fat was accumulating around his mid-section was causing a lot of stress on his joints and lower back – where he developed a bulging disk due to his weight.

When Bill started exercising with me, he couldn't perform many basic tests or exercises due to his weight and bulging disk. Since he couldn't perform many exercise tests a client of even average ability would use to pre-test, I did two things. First, I asked him what his lower back pain was on a scale of 1-10 (10 being the worst pain) every day. He started the first week at a consistent "8". The second thing we did to keep things simple was a timed 1-mile walk to measure his progress. Unfortunately, about 300 meters into the mile, he had to stop because the pain in his back was so severe (which I had no idea was hindering him to that extent before we started). After experiencing the realization that he couldn't walk even a half-mile without stopping, he was ready to make some major changes.

I gave Bill a basic program to follow that included exercises for the entire body performed three times per week, with core exercises and stretches performed on the same days and lower back stretches performed six days per week. The only core exercises we did were front and side planks on the knees, hip bridges, and bird-dog. The lower back stretches were done while lying on his back and utilizing a physioball. His diet only changed slightly, mainly focusing on decreasing the amount of bread he was eating (he had 6-10 pieces of bread a day), drinking more water and leaving everything else the same.

After 8 weeks, Bill's lower back pain changed from an "8" to a "2", with his back rarely hurting at all as to prevent him from performing any daily activities. His strength, endurance, blood glucose, weight and mindset all improved. He was now on the fast track to getting his health back, all thanks to a little bit of exercise and one minor change in his diet.

Examples of Training Types

Most of these examples don't include core/ab exercises (although the workouts will still strengthen your core), which can be done after completing the given workout or incorporated into the workout.

Circuit Training

Circuit #1: Body Weight

Perform each exercise in a row for 30 seconds each, just resting enough to get set up for the next exercise. Once you perform all exercises in the set, rest 1-2 minutes and repeat 2-4 times.

1. Jump squat/body weight squat
2. Push up
3. Jumping lunge/reverse lunge
4. Front plank
5. Burpee
6. Lateral lunge
7. X-body mountain climbers

Circuit #2: Free Weights

*Know what your 12 RM (a weight with which you can perform 12 reps of the exercise) for each exercise is before you begin (if you don't know what it is beforehand, do a set or two of each exercise to figure out how much weight you should be lifting).

Perform 8-10 reps of each exercise (in this situation, since you are doing this as a circuit, only performing 8-10 reps with your 12 RM is OK) and rest just enough (5-10 seconds) between exercises to get set up for the next one. Once you get through the circuit of exercises, rest 2-3 minutes and repeat 2-4 times.

1. Goblet squat
2. Dumbbell bench press
3. Dumbbell bent over row
4. Dumbbell step up

5. Dumbbell shoulder press
6. Dumbbell bicep curl
7. Dumbbell overhead tricep extension

Supersets

Workout #1: My Design

Using your 12 RM, perform exercises 1a and 1b back-to-back with no rest in between, rest 10-30 seconds, and repeat until you've performed your prescribed number of sets of each pair of exercises (between 2-4 sets). Then rest again 10-30 seconds and perform exercises 2a and 2b back-to-back, and so forth until you've completed all supersets.

    1a.   Barbell bench press
    1b.   Seated row

    2a.   Back squat
    2b.   Arnold press

    3a.   Lat pulldown
    3b.   Dips/assisted dip machine

    4a.   Dumbbell walking lunge
    4b.   Incline dumbbell chest fly

    5a.   Hammer curl
    5b.   Cable tricep pushdown

Workout #2: Your Design

Use the same instructions as "Workout #1" but insert your own exercises. (Example: Push: shoulder press, Pull: lat pulldown)

    1a.   Lower body:
    1b.   Upper body push:

    2a.   Upper body pull:
    2b.   Upper body push:

    3a.   Lower body:
    3b.   Upper body pull:

4a. Upper body push:
4b. Lower body:

5a. Core:
5b. Upper body pull:

Compound Sets

Beginning with your 12 RM, perform each pair of exercises (1a/1b) back-to-back, with no rest in between. Rest for 10-30 seconds before moving onto the next set (2a/2b). After completing all pairs, rest 2-3 minutes and repeat 2-4 times.

*You likely won't be able to always do the same number of reps on the 2nd exercise of each pair, and that is A-Okay.

1a. Back squat
1b. Dumbbell step up

2a. Barbell bench press
2b. Cable chest fly

3a. Barbell bent over row
3b. DB reverse fly

4a. Dips/assisted dips
4b. Tricep pushdown

5a. Barbell/EZ bar bicep curl
5b. DB hammer curl

*Notice that the first of the two exercises is more complex, or requires more muscle mass to perform, when there is a reasonable difference between the exercises.

Pre-Exhaustion

Remember, this technique is for those who are accustomed to resistance training and have perfected the technique of all involved exercises. I don't advise training this way if you have been resistance training regularly for less than one year.

Perform your 12RM of each exercise pair (1a/1b) back-to-back, with no rest in between. Rest for 10-30 seconds and move onto 2a/2b. After completing all pairs, rest 2-3 minutes and repeat 2-4 times.

When doing this type of training, it is also common for all prescribed sets to be completed on each pair of exercises or each muscle group before moving to the next pair. With the same exercises listed below, you could perform 3 sets of 1a/1b with 30-90 seconds rest between sets, and then move onto performing 3 sets of 2a/2b, etc.

1a. Leg extension
1b. Front squat

2a. Cable fly
2b. Dumbbell bench press

3a. Hamstring curl
3b. Dumbbell walking lunge

4a. Reverse fly
4b. Seated row

5a. Dumbbell tricep kickback
5b. Dips/assisted dips

Power Training

Perform each exercise until all 3 sets are complete. Notice the rest periods for each exercise. I recommend adding kettlebell swings (only if you've perfected the form) to your warm up before beginning the workout to better prepare the lower body for the powerful movements required and the triple-extension/hip hinge movement of extending the hips, knees and ankles required by most power lifts.

1. Power cleans: 3 x 5
   Rest 3 mins between sets
   *If you haven't done this exercise before, have a qualified coach or trainer instruct you how to do so.

2. 1-arm dumbbell snatch: 3 x 5
   Rest 2-3 mins between sets
   *If you haven't done this exercise before, have a qualified coach or trainer instruct you how to do so.

3. Power/clap push-ups: 3 x failure (technique fails to stay correct or your hands don't leave the ground)
   Rest 2-3 mins between sets

4. Forward med ball slams: 3 x 6
   Rest 60 seconds between sets

5. Lateral med ball toss (both directions = 1 set): 3 x 6
   Rest 60 seconds between sets

If you're new to exercising, new to resistance training, or just don't recognize the names of certain exercises that are included in my examples above, please visit:

https://lifetimelean.com/learn/instruction/

Here, you will find detailed video and written instruction, common tips, and the difficulty of certain exercises. Even if you think you have something down because you've "done it before", feel free to refresh yourself and *make sure* you're performing the exercises as I intend.

These exercises are a starting point. There are hundreds of exercises out there that can be discovered and might be more appealing or effective than some of the ones I've provided instruction for. I urge you to find exercises that you enjoy doing and that you can perform safely.

Finding a program or set of exercises you like doing can take some time, so don't give in after only trying a few different combinations. Once you become more experienced, I encourage you to try each of the workouts given above to see how you like them (with Pre-Exhaustion being the last one you try after gaining enough experience). If you have the option, have a qualified fitness professional watch you perform the exercises to make sure you're doing them correctly.

Diet

"The only real mistake is the one from which we learn nothing."
-Henry Ford

Where to Begin

Health is essentially a game of guess-and-check; each person is different, and your diet might arguably be the biggest factor in the game. We all know that crash-dieting usually doesn't work in the long term and that it's more likely to do more harm than good - even if you look good for that one week of vacation before you pile the weight back on.

I want to help you change your behaviors by *really* taking an in-depth look at your diet and some of your eating-related lifestyle habits. Changing your behaviors, rather than just the number of calories you may restrict yourself down to in order to lose weight, has been shown to keep the weight off in the long run far better than a crash diet that might yield greater short-term results (1, 2, 24).

The other strategies in this book can also be described as a game of guess-and-check, because what I or anyone else can tell you is that everyone is different and guessing and checking how your body is impacted by a certain "health tip" is the easiest way to find out what works for you. The body will react in different ways to different stimuli; and no person's body will react to every food the same as any other one person's body.

While figuring out what types of foods work best for you and at what times, it will help to track what you eat. If you already know what works best for you (or know your own food allergies and sensitivities, how many calories and macros you consume each day, etc.) and you can maintain your current goal body composition without undue effort, then disregard that step because you're awesome and everyone wants to be more like you (*air-five*).

Depending on your allergies, food sensitivities and gut as a whole, eating the same pre-workout meal, post-workout meal, snack or breakfast as your friend might have totally different consequences for you. You might love snacking on raw broccoli and hummus and it may even make you feel good. Your buddy might eat two pieces of raw broccoli and be bloated and burping for the next 45 minutes. This is one small example of many that can be easily spotted and that displays the interpersonal differences that are present inside of us.

What I'm trying to get at is that following the same diet as someone you know because it's "healthier" may or may not yield the same results. Trying things on your own is a must.

Eating "health foods" such as avocado or flaxseed for satiety and quality micro- and macronutrients should, of course, have a similar benefit to your body as it does someone else's, but to expect to be able to eat the same amount of those foods and at the same periods of time for the same exact results is foolish.

The amount of fat, protein, fiber, vitamins and minerals in one serving of these foods will play a smaller part of a day's worth of eating for a 200-lb active male than it will for a 120-lb sedentary female.

If the male in this situation was used to consuming 4 Tbsp. of ground flaxseed throughout the day and told his 120-lb female friend to *eat a couple Tbsp. of flax in the morning, it'll totally help you stay satisfied till lunch time* because it's "healthy" for him, would likely result in an upset digestive system for the female and a lot of time sitting on the porcelain throne. Your diet is going to be different in a variety of ways from everyone else's diet. Part of the diet puzzle is figuring out which foods make you feel good and which foods make you feel like crap.

If you've ever been on any diet or "health kick" for longer than a few weeks, you probably have experienced this first hand:

You're feeling great. You've consumed less sugar, drank less coffee, eaten more vegetables and exercised an extra two hours per week. Then you decide, *ehh, a small fry, soda and double cheeseburger won't kill me*, so you stop in the drive-thru on the way home from work. You're right, it won't kill you. But 1-2 hours later you find yourself feeling sluggish and craving more junk food; and so the cycle begins again.

If you've been in this situation, it's a very good thing to be aware of. When you eat well, you feel well and often times it encourages and motivates you to continue eating well. When you eat junk food sporadically enough in between decent bouts of healthy eating, it makes it more obvious that your body is telling you it doesn't like to function on what you just fed it. Keep your eyes (and your stomach) on this feeling the next time you decide to have a little (or big) treat. The more you recognize it, the better your chances of remembering what you felt like the last time you slipped up a little too much, and the better your chances are of choosing a better option instead.

If you're one to have a "treat meal" now and then (I mean, who doesn't – but our definitions of "now and then" are likely all over the place), having treat meals doesn't inherently need to be the worst food you can find to kill a craving and make that treat meal "worth it". To be able to have a treat meal and *not* feel like complete crap for a few hours afterward should be a superpower. If you have that superpower, keep it up. If you don't, try toning back your next treat meal and see how your body responds.

I believe the secret to finding lasting and sustainable health when it comes to eating is to be able to eat healthy enough that you are able to *listen* to your body, make adjustments, and maintain that type of diet, whatever it is, without undue effort (like always recording everything, measuring/weighing food, counting calories, etc.) and while maintaining a body composition that you're happy with.

Examples of a body that *can't* inform its owner with correct hunger signals would be: thinking you're hungry when you're just dehydrated and need to drink water; craving high-carb snacks/junk food (resulting from eating those foods in the first place, which are very void of nutrients) when you've already eaten more than enough calories in a day; frequently having periods of low energy and high energy throughout the day; and even just feeling unsatisfied after eating an entire meal. If you've experienced any or all of those situations, you may have some work to do.

On the other hand, when you drink enough water and consume a sufficient amount of macronutrients and micronutrients from whole foods, your body has the natural ability to tell you when it's hungry and what it's hungry for (assuming your hormones aren't out of whack). It can give you signals that will make it clear what foods make you feel good and what (hopefully, less frequently eaten) junk foods make you feel lethargic, bloated and/or craving more junk food. Recognizing those types of signals will help you feel more in-tune with your own body and it'll allow you to stay on track long term. One reason I've seen crash diets fail so often is that people will just blindly follow advice they're told will help them lose weight or reach whatever goal they're after, taking no time to be mindful and soak up the experience. I'll dig into this later and give you some tips and guidelines that I, along with my clients, follow that I believe work pretty well.

What I would like to point out to you is a list of the "good" and the "bad" in your diet through a 3-day dietary recall (by the way, I don't condone regularly labeling foods as "good" or "bad", but for this exercise we're going to talk about them that way). By looking at what you eat after having it written down, it usually becomes apparent where you're lacking and what foods you're eating too much of.

Start out by tracking what you eat for 3 days, including one weekend day. I've also provided a few extra blank days in case you want to track more. You're going to look at what meal/snack you were eating (breakfast, afternoon snack, etc.), the food you consumed (double cheese-burger, carrots, etc.), where you got the food (home-grown, Burger King, grocery store, etc.), the amount you ate (1 cup, 2 pieces, etc.), the time of day you ate (6:00am, etc.), how you were feeling at the time (hungry, sad, angry, bored, anxious, stressed, etc.), what activity you engaged in before or after eating (post-3 mile run, none, etc.), and maybe most importantly, *why* you chose the food you ate (healthy, unhealthy, convenient, it jumped into my mouth without me knowing it, etc.). These tables will give you a lot of insight into your own diet and your diet habits you probably haven't thought about before. Notice how I leave *plenty* of room to include more than just three meals per day (let's not kid ourselves).

Weekday 1: Mon Tues Wed Thurs (circle)

Meal/ Snack	Food	Food Source	Amount	Time of day	Feelings at that time	Activity before/ After	Why you chose that food

Table 2.1

Weekday 2: Mon Tues Wed Thurs (circle)

Meal/ Snack	Food	Food Source	Amount	Time of day	Feelings at that time	Activity before/ After	Why you chose that food

Table 2.2

Weekday 3: Mon Tues Wed Thurs (circle)

Meal/ Snack	Food	Food Source	Amount	Time of day	Feelings at that time	Activity before/ After	Why you chose that food

Table 2.3

Weekday 4: Mon Tues Wed Thurs (circle)

Meal/ Snack	Food	Food Source	Amount	Time of day	Feelings at that time	Activity before/ After	Why you chose that food

Table 2.4

Weekend Day 1: Fri Sat Sun (circle)

Meal/ Snack	Food	Food Source	Amount	Time of day	Feelings at that time	Activity before/ After	Why you chose that food

Table 2.5

Weekend Day 2: Fri Sat Sun (circle)

Meal/ Snack	Food	Food Source	Amount	Time of day	Feelings at that time	Activity before/ After	Why you chose that food

Table 2.6

Weekend Day 3: Fri Sat Sun (circle)

Meal/ Snack	Food	Food Source	Amount	Time of day	Feelings at that time	Activity before/ After	Why you chose that food

Table 2.7

Now that you have a place to track and further examine your eating habits and refer to later on, I want to talk about some of the problems and solutions that I believe should be addressed when it comes to eating.

The Who, What, When, Where, Why, and How of Your Diet

Who

The who I want to discuss includes you and your family, and sometimes your friends and coworkers. This includes anyone involved in the shopping, choosing, cooking, or eating process that revolves around your snacks and meals. If I had a dollar (or maybe 20) for every time I heard someone say, "Well, I usually eat pretty healthy but my *insert husband/wife/friend/boss* is the one who chooses/influences what I eat most of the time", I could've retired before I had the chance to finish this book.

Just like the control you have over your physical activity or whether you make time to be active each day (or at least consistently each week), you control what goes into your mouth; unless you're a newborn baby, and in that case I don't think you'd be reading this right now. The excuses you keep telling yourself for why you haven't made any positive changes in your diet are running out.

The good news is, I know what it's like to be the only one seemingly fighting everyone else to maintain a healthy diet. Almost every single day I'm asked or told to just "live a little and have some" or something along those lines in almost every situation I'm in. A majority of my friends in college could've cared less about exercise, eating a healthy diet, or consuming less alcohol. As you could imagine, every weekend was a battle to stay on track if I were spending any time being social. If I listened to every offer I got to eat something I wouldn't normally eat, I'd probably be 30+ pounds overweight right now.

The people around you can influence what you eat, no doubt about it. What needs to change, and strengthen, is your willpower and wisdom to say "no thanks".

For example, if you enjoyed exercising every day because you like the way it makes you feel and you know it's good for you, would you skip the gym every time someone said, "Hey, come sit and watch a movie with me, you don't need to work out tonight"? Sooner than you expect, those skipped workouts will start to add up, just as accepting someone else's unhealthy food choices and habits now and again will add up day after day, week after week until you look back and realize what you've been eating the past 3 months and suddenly you've gained 10 pounds.

I'm not saying don't treat yourself (I'll get to that later) or be deathly afraid of missing one workout, but there needs to be *some* level of self-control in those situations. Those who have social support on any fitness or diet endeavor almost always have an easier time making it last. Those who don't have social support and are constantly battling friends, family and coworkers about their exercise or diet habits or have no support whatsoever are the people who usually fall off course.

Solution

The best way to involve those around you who have been more of a negative influence on your diet than a positive one is to tell them why you're choosing what you are, even if they don't understand it at first. Tell your family or friends you want to or need to lose some weight because you just went in for a check-up and you have higher cholesterol and blood pressure than you prefer. Tell them you want to have stronger bones and joints so you can stay injury-free and active later in life. Making it personal will help others see the reason you're making these choices and hopefully help them support you as well.

Obviously, having healthier food in the house for breakfast and dinner requires effort from the entire family because they likely will have to eat that healthier food as well. It's pretty easy to buy healthy and unhealthy food options when shopping and think to yourself that you'll choose the healthy one at home and the kids will get Captain Crunch like they wanted, but sometimes things don't go as planned. When the worse option is there, more often than not (at least in the beginning) that's what is going to be chosen over the healthier option while you're learning new eating habits.

Having a talk with your family about what types of foods are going to be in the house can increase the likelihood of staying on track longer. That way, everyone can still have some of what they enjoy splurging on but also eat a majority of the foods we know are going to improve our health.

The same situation applies to friends and coworkers. If the guys or girls like to go out on Friday night and have drinks at a bar, by all means enjoy your night out guilt-free if that's something you really enjoy. When those same people order in fast food or greasy Chinese for lunch 5 days per week and ask if you want to add to their order, that's when the opportunity to make a consistent healthy decision arises. Those seemingly harmless lunches, since you still may have a chance for a healthy dinner, will start to add up, and by failing to plan, you're planning to fail. If you know you're going to be around someone or some situation where you're almost certainly going to be tempted by unhealthy choices, have a plan and stick to it.

There are a few other strategies that I've found success with when dealing with those negative influences around you at social events, family gatherings, or holidays.

- Tell them your goals and why what they're pressuring on you isn't going to get you closer to reaching them. Divert the attention off of you and onto them by asking if they have any health/fitness/body composition goals they're striving for. Maybe you'll get them to put the cake down, and maybe you'll make a new friend who has similar goals as you but just doesn't have anyone to support them yet either.

- Use the "next time" or "yesterday" excuse. When turning someone down who just won't leave you alone, it works quite well to either tell them, "Sorry I'll have to pass today, but maybe next time I will." Or tell them, "I shouldn't have any more of that, I ate a bunch of *insert junk food here* yesterday." Whether you actually plan on having some next time or actually ate that certain food yesterday doesn't matter; what does matter is that person is now off your back about what you're choosing to eat at the time because since you've already eaten it, they can now feel better about themselves eating it too.

- Do your best not to draw attention to yourself or anyone else's dish. The less comments you make about other peoples' food, the less likely they are to comment on yours. When I was first diving into the nutrition world (and when I wasn't *nearly* as wise), I was sometimes that annoying person pointing out what my friends and family were eating. Now I know how annoying it can be when it happens to me and I don't do it nearly as often to others, if at all, unless I know that person wants me to point it out or they want me to give them my opinion on said food.

Don't be afraid to let people in on your health choices. If they have no idea why you're choosing to do what you are, telling them why it's important to you might be all you need to do to get them off your back; or maybe even supporting you.

What

Your "diet" is simply what you eat. So yes, you're always on a "diet". Most people hear the word diet and think of cutting calories, not eating carbs, not having any more sugared beverages, and so on. I won't tell you exactly how much to eat of which foods to get the recommended amount of macronutrients or micronutrients for your body weight, goals and activity level because I don't think that's the most important aspect of learning better eating habits. I want to focus on the basics and the main influences on a "good" or a "bad" diet. Later on, I'll provide you with a simple foundation for a grocery list you can try to incorporate into your daily diet and see how those foods make you feel.

One hot topic I'd like to address before getting into the *"what"* of diet is fiber consumption. I recommend consuming approximately 40g and 30g of fiber per day for men and women, respectively. I know that's above the current recommendations (and is dependent upon the individual), but I know from experience that hitting fiber goals is one of the most elusive accomplishments our dieting population strives for.

When I recommend that amount of fiber to *work up to,* I know most people will have a hard time hitting it every single day (this is almost always the case with getting enough protein as well). I would prefer you aim for a few grams higher each day because more often than not life takes over and busy schedules lead to imperfect diets, and imperfect diets are frequently the ones lacking in fiber.

If you eat 2 servings less of veggies, one serving less of fruit, and one serving less of complex carbs than you planned on any given day, you'd likely be 10-15 grams below your fiber goal - it's that easy. Aiming high can give you some leeway in case you don't eat exactly what you planned. Trust me, if you eat the right amount of fruits and vegetables every day, consume complex carbs such as oats or quinoa, and have healthy snacks like nuts and seeds, these recommendations will be a piece of cake (which does *not* contain much fiber).

As you're increasing your fiber intake, like with the example of the 120-lb female, be sure to do so *slowly*, and work up to the daily recommendation if you're not quite there yet. Pay attention to the signals your body is giving you. If you mistakenly end up constipated (or the opposite), ease back on the amount of fiber you try to consume in a day and go from there.

Fiber is not only important for regular bowel movements, but a majority of evidence has also shown that fiber can normalize bowel movements, maintain bowel health, lower cholesterol, help control blood sugar levels, increase satiety and help individuals maintain a healthy weight. Consuming a healthy amount of fiber may also decrease the risk of cardiovascular disease, high blood pressure, diabetes, inflammation, obesity and certain types of cancer (3-6).

The great thing about consciously consuming enough fiber each day is that by getting your fiber intake from whole foods (rather than a supplement), you're automatically going to be eating healthier on a consistent basis without having to obsess over what types or what amounts of food you're eating. Fiber intake goes hand-in-hand with beginning to eat a healthier diet that includes the right whole grains, fats, fruits and vegetables each day. Just be wary of looking for packaged foods that boast *"high in fiber!"* to meet your daily amount – they can be a good thing at the start, but also pose the risk of reinforcing the idea of getting important nutrients from man-made foods instead of the real deal.

If you have trouble getting enough veggies in each day, try strategies such as putting leafy greens and other fairly flavorless varieties of veggies in smoothies, soups, and chili (yes, even if the recipe doesn't call for them). Add raw or frozen leafy greens into your scrambled eggs and cook them until they're wilted, so they're less noticeable and you don't feel like you're eating a handful of leaves with your eggs. Or ask your friends how they get creative with vegetables. I know I can get bored of plain raw veggies once in a while, so do what you can to try different options until you find some you enjoy.

The modern diet we have come to know and love has been described as the "Western" diet (7). This type of diet is often just devoid of nutrient-dense foods and high in processed carbs, fried foods, liquid calories and sugar. This is the type of diet that can lead to very preventable diseases such as type II diabetes, metabolic disease, heart disease, hypertension, and hyperlipidemia.

Not to scare you or anything, but diabetes (specifically type II diabetes) is one of the most preventable and dangerous diseases of our time. Many people in the US (diagnosed and undiagnosed) have the precursor to the full-blown disease, known as prediabetes, and you may be one of them without even knowing it.

From 2005-2008, 35% of US adults 20 years or older had prediabetes, and that increases to 50% of adults 65 years and older. In 2009-2012, those numbers increased to 37% and 51%, respectively. Diabetes is the leading cause of kidney failure, non-traumatic lower-limb amputations, and blindness among US adults. It is also a major cause of heart disease and stroke as well as the 7th leading cause of death in the US (8, 9). This disease can sneak up on you before you even know you're prediabetic - and suddenly you could go in for a routine physical and be diagnosed with diabetes (10). In all age categories by 2012, a scary 27.8% of people with diabetes were undiagnosed (9). The worst part about this disease is that it's one of the most preventable diseases of our time – through a decent diet and consistent exercise.

That's not all. If you like money and time and want more of both, consider this: a 2014 review looking at the impact of lifestyle intervention on obese adults with type II diabetes found that over 10 years, those with basic but regular lifestyle intervention had fewer medications, lower health-care costs, and fewer hospitalizations. They also saved an average of $5,280 over a 10-year period compared to the group without lifestyle intervention (11). That's $5,280 you'd have to spend on your home, kids, hobbies or healthier food – all brought to you by some regular exercise, a diet that meets (or gets close to meeting because nobody is perfect) the recommendations, and a little extra social support and disease education.

As a kid, I was on the fast track to poor health as an adult with the way I ate. I always wanted the extra serving, the biggest piece of dessert and the tastiest snacks I could get my hands on. As you already know, or will soon find out, the process of changing eating habits must be gradual if it's going to stick. But what anyone who has gone through a drastic health transformation (whether it's physical, psychological, or emotional) can tell you is that it's *always* worth it once it becomes easy to maintain and it lasts.

This is what a typical day of eating for me as a young high school student would look like:

Breakfast

2 bowls of cereal (Honey Bunches of Oats, Captain Crunch, Fruity Pebbles, etc.)
1 bagel w/ cream cheese or peanut butter
1-2 C apple juice
1 banana
1 orange
1 yogurt
1 C water

Mid-Morning Snack

1 granola bar (if I had anything, but usually I didn't)
2 C water

Lunch

2 servings of whatever school lunch was having (didn't matter, I'd eat it)
1 serving of fruit
Maybe 1 serving of vegetables
1 nutty bar
1 chocolate milk
2 C water

Mid-Afternoon Snack

Graham cracker ice cream sandwich or
Little Debbies like Swiss Cake Rolls or Zebra Cakes
Maybe some Skippy peanut butter on a banana
4 C water

Dinner

3 C mac & cheese, extra cheese
½ C Peanuts
1 serving canned or frozen veggies
1 hot dog in the mac & cheese
1 apple

1 can of Mountain Dew
3 C water

<u>Snack</u>

1 bowl of ice cream <u>or</u>
Peanut butter toast with banana on top
3 C water

    I hope you're thinking what I'm thinking; that was kind of a disaster. The sad thing is, most of the high school students I coach or work with eat similar to this or worse. Only a handful of athletes I know of eat a fairly healthy diet throughout high school.

    I want you to rate that diet on a scale of 1-10, with "1" being absolute worst, and "10" being absolute best where nothing needs to be changed, and remember that number.

This is what I basically eat on a daily basis now:

<u>"Tuesday"</u>

5:45am: 20oz cool water, 2/3 C Oats w/ a banana, 1 Tbsp. of ground flax seed, cinnamon, 1-2 Tbsp. natural PB, half a scoop of whey protein. Four eggs cooked in olive or coconut oil w/ turmeric, basil, oregano, thyme, black pepper, and/or cilantro w/ occasional 1-2 slices of turkey or ham and 2 cups spinach with salsa and optional avocado (if I eat this and don't have oats or it's post-workout, I make it into a breakfast burrito with 1 wrap w/ ~6g/protein, 7g/fiber, and 25g/carbs per wrap).

~10am: 20oz water. Smoothie – 1 C unsweetened almond milk, 1 tsp chia seeds, 1 tsp PB, 1 cup frozen kale or spinach, 3/4 cup frozen berries, 1 scoop whey protein. Handful of cocoa covered almonds and handful of cereal. <u>OR</u>
2/3 C plain Greek yogurt, 1 scoop whey protein, 1 Tbsp. chia seeds, 1 banana or 1/4 C berries, 1 Tbsp. PB, cinnamon.

11am: 10oz water. Workout: ~45 minutes weight lifting, 10 minutes stair stepping or rowing.

1pm: 20oz water. 2 chicken breasts cooked in ~1 Tbsp. olive or coconut oil seasoned with whatever I feel like (same seasonings as above or lemon/pepper seasoning) and 1 whole bag (~4 servings) of frozen mixed veggies with olive oil and garlic with some optional parmesan cheese on top, 1 apple.

1-6pm: 30-40oz water. 1 handful of strawberries. 1 handful of almonds.

6pm: ~9oz Salmon with variety of seasonings on top, sautéed peppers, mushrooms, onions in 1 tsp. olive or coconut oil, and a sweet potato with hummus. If I've got it, maybe a couple bites of vanilla ice cream as well.

8pm: 20oz water. If I didn't eat the Greek yogurt mixture earlier in the day, I'd have that now, or 2/3 C cottage cheese and a small handful of walnuts and/or raisins.

Now rate my diet on a scale of 1-10 just like you did before. Look at the amount and frequency of water consumption, the planning of meals (often times prepared in advance), my protein intake, the extra ingredients I add to my cooking and the amount of fruits and veggies I fit in each day. What was the difference between the two? I'd imagine (if you've paid attention) there's a drastic difference between the two ratings you've given me.

Obviously, this is going to look different because being in high school doesn't give you the opportunity to make great snacks (like a smoothie mid-morning) or cook your own lunch. There's not much kids can do about that. It's breakfast, snacking, and dinner that really provide an important opportunity to get kids eating better foods.

Don't expect to change your diet like I did over the course of a couple months and have it stick. This was years of learning, failing, succeeding, failing and learning again. It's not about quick progress. It's about lasting progress. If you've lost weight before but gained it all back, I'm not impressed, and you shouldn't be either. I want to see the "before and *second* after" photo (the photo taken 6-12+ months *after* your health-kick ended), not just the "before and after" photo.

If you don't follow what I mean, take this example: A woman comes in to meet with me about changing her diet and lifestyle habits. She shows me this impressive "before and after" photo that was taken two years ago. She doesn't exactly look the same as the "after" photo anymore, but the transformation was impressive.

I ask, *"So, what have you done in the past to try to lose weight? And did it work?"*

She says, *"Well, I've tried this diet… and that diet… and this one diet worked really well, actually. It kind of forced me to write down what I ate so I had a general idea of how many calories I was eating each day. I lost like 30 pounds the first 2 months."*

I respond with, *"Okay, but how well did that diet really work?"*

After it dawns on her, she realizes that diet must *not* have worked that well, since in fact she is back in this situation again. *Oh… never mind.*

You shouldn't *need* to count calories to "succeed" or follow a special diet for the rest of your life to maintain your weight. For most people, it can be quite simple, for example: focus on eating protein at each meal and snack (size of your palm); get at least 3-5 servings of veggies of various colors in per day (size of your closed fist); eat an average of 2-3 servings of fruit of various colors if possible per day (size of your cupped hand); eat 3-6 servings of complex carbs per day (size of your cupped hand); and eat 3-5 servings of healthy fats per day (size of your thumb).

With each balanced meal, your general goal could be to consume one serving of each of these if you're a female. Men could (and depending on how active you are and if you resistance train) consume the same but with an extra serving of protein, veggies, fats, and carbs at each main meal (12).

If there was a diet generalization that I found to be very true just based on observations, it would be that people who eat enough protein for their activity level and goals and who eat more vegetables than the average person end up being the leanest. Don't take this the wrong way because there are no absolutes in this area, but looking at diet simply, the more vegetables and protein a person eats, the leaner they tend to be.

Of course, you can't just live off vegetables, which is why it's important to have good sources of protein (whether animals or plants) at each meal/snack and healthy fats every day, but the veggies are more important than people realize – they're full of fiber, they're nutrient-dense, they're not calorie-dense, they take up a lot of space in your stomach, and they're packed with micronutrients, phytochemicals and antioxidants that you don't usually get from eating processed foods. Naturally, the more of those that you eat, the easier time you'll have staying lean or losing weight (as long as you *enjoy* eating them and cooking them in different ways).

There are, of course, some exceptions to this. If you're an athlete or simply very active, you may need to consume more carbs than described for each meal. If you're sedentary and don't tolerate carbs very well, you may only want to consume 2 servings of complex carbs per day and save those for breakfast, lunch, and/or post-workout. As you should know by now, there is too much variability between individuals to give a "perfect" recommendation. The advice I've given thus far is simply to keep you thinking about eating a balanced diet each day, to ensure that you don't need to be obsessive about tracking everything you eat to make progress, and to make you aware of your eating as to not become deficient in any one category.

Why You Should (Usually) Avoid Drinking Your Calories

I believe liquid calorie consumption is one of the leading causes of the obesity epidemic we're currently sitting in (pun intended). Those who consume many of their extra and unnecessary calories each day from liquids tend to be overweight more often than those who don't consume an equal amount of calories from liquids (again, based off my own observations of people across various age groups). Though the reason isn't the liquid calories themselves, it's how they fit into a person's diet.

Do you remember the last time you just couldn't help yourself and overate on raw veggies, unsalted almonds or baked fish? There probably hasn't been a time because that's near impossible unless you're force-feeding yourself.

The reason liquid calories are so easy to overdue is because of how easy it is to consume large amounts of calories and not feel satisfied afterwards. You can consume 400 liquid calories in a matter of seconds and still want more while the same amount in veggies and lean protein is going to fill you up every single time, and take 10x as long to consume.

Some of the worst culprits for excessive liquid calorie consumption, as I mentioned earlier, are flavored coffee drinks (1-2 cups of regular coffee is A-Okay in my book), sports drinks, energy drinks, fruit juices, alcohol, and, of course, soda.

There is research to prove the negative consequences of consuming liquid calories. Researchers had subjects consume one meal per week with no beverage or a beverage of equal volume containing 0 calories or ~156 calories. Subjects who consumed a beverage containing calories ended up consuming 104 more calories on average per meal than those who drank a calorie-free beverage; and those who drank the 100+ extra calories at each meal felt no more satisfied than those who drank 0 calories (13). This is just one example, but there are many more examples of the benefits of being properly hydrated with water when it comes to weight maintenance, weight loss, and disease prevention (14-16). By all means, have some liquid calories in moderation if you really enjoy them, but if you consume some of these more than a few times per week and wonder why you struggle to lose weight or stay satisfied, the answer is pretty clear.

Some of the better liquid calorie options that actually can offer some health benefit include, but are not limited to, coffee (with creamer to make it actually have a somewhat substantial number of calories), milk, unsweetened almond/coconut milk and low-calorie or calorie-free electrolyte beverages for athletes. When consuming these products, it's still always going to be wise to check how many calories are in each serving and how many servings you're accustomed to drinking each day (so you can keep calorie consumption in check with liquids) along with the ingredient list.

If you're an athlete of some sort, consuming a beverage with added carbohydrates and electrolytes during/between competitions of greater than 90 minutes doesn't necessarily apply to what is stated above. Carbohydrate and electrolyte consumption during prolonged activity can help sustain performance as well as help prevent dehydration and muscle cramps – it's when people get used to drinking sports drinks with 200+ calories per bottle at times when their body doesn't need the energy that they may run into issues.

As you can imagine, water should pretty much always be your #1 beverage choice. Cutting out liquid calories, or at least cutting back on them, can help you lose weight and control your weight loss with ease. As a general recommendation, aim to drink half of your bodyweight (in pounds) in ounces of water per day. That means if you weigh 200 lbs, drink around 100 ounces of water per day. If you exercise and/or sweat a lot, that number should increase to account for body water lost through sweat. If you don't exercise or sweat a lot, sorry, but that number can still be your goal. Once you start drinking more water each day, inevitably you're going to have to use the restroom more than you're used to. Don't worry, that will fade slightly, just like getting sore after beginning to resistance train will decrease as well.

If you consider my recommendations (these aren't new either) and eat mostly real, unprocessed foods and follow the "hand-sized" serving sizes described earlier, you shouldn't have to stress about counting calories or adding up grams of fiber.

Below is a list of simple food swaps that can increase your intake of quality macronutrients, micronutrients, vitamins, minerals and/or fiber.

Food Substitutes

1. Sweet potatoes for baked potatoes (both have very similar macros, though)
2. Spaghetti squash for spaghetti noodles
3. Oats for cereal
4. Almond/cashew/sunflower butter for peanut butter (natural – peanuts and salt – peanut butter is still OK by me)
5. Spinach/kale/arugula for iceberg/romaine lettuce
6. Quinoa for spaghetti noodles
7. Avocado/plain Greek yogurt for mayonnaise
8. Plain Greek yogurt for sour cream
9. Plain Greek yogurt w/ flavored whey protein for pre-made flavored yogurt varieties
10. Almond or coconut milk (preferably unsweetened) for cow's milk
11. Olive/coconut/avocado oil for vegetable/soybean/safflower/palm oil
12. Homemade popcorn with real butter for chips/store bought popcorn
13. Hummus for generic sour cream-based chip/veggie dip

To give you more ideas of some types of mainly real foods you can enjoy daily and what I recommend looking at for ideas when you just don't know what to eat:

Breakfast

100% rolled oats/steel cut oats
    Add-ins: honey (post-workout), **PB, almond butter, flax seed, chia seeds, hemp seeds,** dark chocolate chips, berries, banana, cinnamon, **walnuts,** etc. Add ≥1 type of good **fat** to it
Kashi GoLean Cereals (<6g sugar per serving)
Eggs on whole-wheat English muffin
Breakfast burrito (homemade) - eggs, veggies, salsa, hummus, etc.
Scrambled eggs in coconut oil with veggies
Hard-boiled eggs and hummus
Turkey bacon
Protein shake/fruit and yogurt smoothie (add a fat like chia seed/ground flaxseed/peanut butter/almond butter)
Fruit/yogurt smoothie/parfait (add in a fat)

Snacks

Almonds, walnuts, pistachios, sunflower seeds, etc.
Veggies with hummus
Fruit with a nut butter/nuts
Protein shake and piece of fruit/made into a smoothie (with added fat)
String cheese/Babybel cheese
Plain Greek yogurt (< 12g sugar per serving) with ground nuts and flavored whey protein
Oikos Greek yogurt (Triple Zero is great)
Turkey/beef jerky (less than 2g sugar per serving, and no added sugar would be best)
Dried edamame
Hard boiled eggs
Cottage cheese

Lunch

Leftovers from dinner the night before
Salad greens (romaine, spinach, kale, etc.) with protein (chicken, tuna, salmon, turkey, etc.)
Fruit of your choice
Tuna/chicken wrap with avocado, hummus and spinach
Avocado
Nuts
Veggies - raw or frozen
Crockpot meals (thrown together at breakfast, ready at lunch or dinner)

Dinner

A protein
A veggie (two servings)
A carb
A fat

Dairy

Milk (almond/coconut milk – says on the label whether it contains calcium or not)
Cheese (in moderation due to ease of over-consumption)
Cottage cheese
Whey/casein protein powders
Butter
Greek yogurt (<12g sugar or plain)
Ice cream/frozen yogurt (mmmmm….. ☺)

Veggies (fresh or frozen)

Broccoli
Asparagus
Greens (spinach, kale, collard greens)
Brussel sprouts
Cauliflower
Green beans
Peas
Bell peppers
Onions
Mushrooms
(Doesn't matter too much – just look for variety)

Fruits

Your choice, but mix it up!
Berries are your best choice when it comes to keeping sugar/calories minimal

Beverages

Water
Coffee (small amount of full-fat/cream is typically better than added sugar or artificial sweeteners)
Tea (*real* tea, not Lipton bottled tea, etc.)
Milk (if you don't get calcium from other sources such as fish, yogurt, some almond/soy milks, cheese, collard greens, etc.)
Alcohol (in moderation! Two drinks a day for men, 1 drink a day for women is recommended maximum)

Fats

Olive/coconut/canola/avocado/sunflower oil
Peanut/almond/cashew/sunflower butter
Avocado
Red meat
Eggs (with the yolk)
Nuts and seeds of any kind (raw/light salt)
Chia/flax/hemp seeds
Salmon/sardines/other fatty fish
Cheese (moderation)
Full fat Greek yogurt
Full fat cottage cheese

Carbs

Quinoa
Buckwheat
Amaranth
Oats
Rice
Brown rice
Brown rice pasta
Black/kidney/white/garbanzo/pinto/etc. beans
Sweet potato/baked potato
Wraps/tortillas (ideally >6g protein and >6g fiber per wrap)
*These are basically all considered "complex carbs"- the slower-digesting and fiber-full versions you want to stick to most of the time. Simple carbs include things like sugars, sweets, soda, fruit juice, cookies, crackers, baked goods, cereals, etc.

Proteins

Chicken breast
Turkey breast/ground turkey
Eggs
Tuna
Salmon
Tilapia
Shellfish

Cod

Pork

Lean red meat (non-lean red meat in moderation, mainly due to calories – a few times per week or less)

Chickpeas

Nuts/seeds

All types of beans

Lentils

Whey/casein protein powder

This fairly short list of foods and meal ideas doesn't include every type of food and combination you can and should eat, it's just a starting point. There are going to be foods on this list that you dislike, and there are going to be foods you don't think you can live without that also aren't on this list.

If you don't already follow some type of grocery list, I encourage you to add and subtract from this list (mindfully, of course) so it's more individualized for you and your lifestyle so you have something to look back to when you're about to go grocery shopping. Like I mentioned before, if you focus on eating whole, unprocessed foods until you're satisfied and not stuffed, you shouldn't need to worry about counting calories. Notice there are some slightly processed foods on this list that aren't single-ingredient items. I'm not going to lie to you and say I never eat anything that isn't processed or that you shouldn't either, because I do, but it's a small amount that isn't on a regular meal-to-meal basis.

If you're wondering what the deal is with *IIFYM* (If It Fits Your Macros, flexible dieting, or some other abbreviated version), that style of eating or dieting requires the minimum of tracking everything you eat and adding up the macronutrients (protein, fats, and carbs) your diet consists of. The main reason most people are not up for this type of dieting is because it takes extra time out of their day and they likely will need a food scale to portion out and weigh the food (in grams) that they're eating to be most accurate.

Those who follow IIFYM or macro counting usually have some type of specific body composition goal in mind when tracking macros. If they're "bulking", you might see a generous increase in carbs and protein and a decrease in fat. If they're "cutting", you might see an increase in protein and fats and a slow decrease in carbs. You might know they own a food scale and hear about how annoying it is to weigh their cup of

Cheerios in the morning, their cut sweet potato for lunch, or their mixed nuts in the evening so they hit their numbers.

You might consistently see them posting pictures of a Pop-Tart-Nutella-peanut butter-ice cream sandwich dipped in chocolate and sprinkles and wonder, *how can they possibly look like that?* Maybe they're a genetic freak who doesn't gain body fat and is simultaneously brain washing everyone who sees it and they believe that it will work for any other Joe-Shmo off the street. Or, maybe those people carefully calculated how many grams of protein, fat, and carbs that abomination (sounds intriguing though, doesn't it?) added to their daily macro intake and it just fit in perfectly. If that treat sounds like something you want to cram into your macros instead of just trying to consistently eat healthy whole foods without tracking calories or macros and then treating yourself occasionally, then consider researching how to "do" IIFYM and give it a try for yourself. It can work wonders on your body composition and physique if you learn how to do it right. If you are completely lost trying this, I would recommend finding someone with solid experience and recommendations and hiring them to coach you through the process.

I don't know everything there is to know on the IIFYM/flexible dieting subject, but I can give you a general idea. When tracking your macronutrients, it's important to know what goal you have in mind and what your body type is. For example, if you're 30 pounds overweight, don't tolerate carbs very well, are sedentary 90% of the day and are interested in fat loss, you're likely going to require less carbs, and more protein and fat than the dietary recommendations you've seen in the past. If you're an endurance runner who's trying to train for an upcoming race or just wants to maintain his/her level of fitness, you're likely going to have a higher proportion of carbs to fuel that activity and a lower proportion of fat (but not for everyone).

Carbs and fat are, for the most part, inversely related. Protein is almost always going to stay around the same 25-35% of daily calories (some people aim higher but it really isn't necessary for the majority), but carbs can fluctuate from the "recommended" ~65% (which I believe, among others, is too high for most people) down to around 30% of daily calories. If you're going to fluctuate your fat calories, be sure to add *healthy* fats to increase that percentage like fatty fish, nuts, seeds, olive/coconut oil, avocado, etc. and not the less-healthy ones like the fats found in baked goods, deep-fried foods, desserts, cookies, chips, and crackers.

The percentage of each macro that you consume can depend on your body type, lean body mass, and goals to name a few. The idea of flexible dieting is to consume mostly healthy whole foods just like every other recommendation, but to be able to do it with the flexibility to eat "bad" foods while staying within your prescribed macros so you can accurately track your progress to meet your goals. Filling up on junk food will waste a lot of your macros and make it very difficult to be satisfied each day, so don't get the idea that you can fit anything into macro numbers you might make up for yourself and still see healthy progress. Find a reliable coach to help you through this until you have a good handle on it.

If you're trying to get leaner, are used to eating a large amount of carbs per day, and want somewhere to start, try aiming for 50% carbs (mostly all whole sources such as quinoa, oats, sweet potatoes, etc.) eaten mostly around your workouts, 25% fat, and 25% protein.

If you're lean and are trying to gain lean muscle mass, try aiming for ~50-60% carbs eaten mostly around your workouts, 30% protein, and 10-20% fat. Those macros can change a lot based on the results you're achieving and the results you want; and they're a *very* general idea of what IIFYM might look like. If you feel lost and haven't been able to see the results you want after many failed attempts (6-8 weeks without seeing your dream physique does not count), it may be wise to consult with a qualified coach, sports nutritionist or dietician.

The total number of calories you consume makes the biggest difference. If you think you're on the right track to losing 0.5 lbs of body fat per week with your current calorie intake and macro split, but you don't see any progress after two weeks of sticking to your diet, then you need to think about adjusting your calorie intake.

An example of an adjustment for this situation might be decreasing the number of calories you get from carbs by 100-150 calories, and decreasing your fat intake by another 100 calories for the next week or two. See progress and don't feel deprived? Then you've found the sweet spot.

A very basic way to determine how many calories you need in a day based on your resting metabolic rate (RMR) is to multiply your body weight in pounds by 10 kcals for women or 11 kcals for men.

This is a daily example of a high-fat macro split for a 203-pound sedentary male using this equation:

203 x 11 = 2,233 kcals

Total kcals to consume to maintain weight: 2,233 kcals

150g protein (600 kcals, 27%), 90g fat (810 kcals, 37%), 200g carbs (800 kcals, 36%) = 2,210 kcals

This individual's calorie intake would change based on his goals. If he were to want to lose 0.5 lbs per week, he'd need to subtract 1,750 kcals per week (in theory, it should take a deficit of ~3500 calories to lose 1 pound) or just 250 kcals per day. He could do that by keeping his diet the exact same, but subtracting 250 kcals from either fat or carbs, or a combination of the two (protein should *at least* stay where it's at if he wants to minimize lean muscle mass loss). If he wanted to just add 30-45 minutes of exercise each day instead, he would likely reach his goal taking that route as well.

There are many different equations out there to calculate how many calories you may need in a day. Some just use body weight, like my example above, and some try to factor in daily activity, occupation, exercise and lean body mass. My best advice to you is either have someone who's qualified (nutritionist, RD, etc.) calculate what you need to eat each day, or take the average RMR calculation from a few different equations, go with that number, and track your progress.

Once again, do your best not to complicate *what* to eat. Remember, crash diets are likely to fail, whole foods are the way to go, and the less processed you eat on a regular basis the easier time you'll have reaching your daily goals of micronutrients and macronutrients.

One last note to keep in mind: tracking your calorie consumption is a useful tool to see where you currently stand, but I don't recommend trying to count calories in the long term. Think about being in a hurry, not weighing your nut butter or salad dressing, and spreading 2 Tbsp. of nut butter on your morning toast or pouring "one" Tbsp. of salad dressing on your salad. Even if you're off by about 1-2 tsp of both each day, that could be a difference of 100-200 calories per day, or 700-1400 calories per week. That could equate to *gaining* or *losing* 0.5-1 lbs every few weeks if you don't closely pay attention to how your body is responding (not to mention, calorie counts on food labels aren't 100% accurate either).

When

When refers to when you eat, plan, or prepare your meals. The best thing you can do to avoid failing is to *plan*. For some, this could be as simple as writing down on the white board calendar in your kitchen what you plan on eating for dinner with your family each night. To make following through with this even easier, decide who's going to prepare it, who's buying the groceries, or even when they need to start preparing it so it fits into everyone's schedule.

Solution

Tools for Staying Prepared

1.   **Invest in a nice Crockpot/slow-cooker.** You put the frozen/uncooked food in while you eat breakfast; it's done when you come home from work. Sprinkle in herbs and spices to change up the taste of similar dishes. Sounds challenging, doesn't it?

2.   **Plan, plan, plan again.** Decide on a time/day, say Sunday afternoon, when you can decide what you're going to eat that week and make sure you have the supplies to prepare it.

3.   **Food preparation.** Some people prepare everything for the week on Sunday and stash it away in the fridge/freezer so it's ready to be taken out when they need it. This can be a bit of an adjustment and seem time consuming for some. If you have extremely busy weekdays but free weekends, this might be for you. If you're not ready for this, try at least cutting up veggies or split healthy snacks such as nuts into plastic bags or Tupperware containers so they're readily available to take out of the house, snack on, or use while cooking meals.

4.   **Grocery shop a day early.** There's nothing setting you up worse to eating fast food for dinner than suddenly noticing you don't have anything to eat in the house. If you wait until your food is completely gone and *then* go grocery shopping, you're likely going to have 1-3 meals that are eaten by scrounging for whatever is collecting dust in the back of your cupboard, not to mention making impulsive decisions on an empty stomach when at the grocery store. Shopping a day

early can guarantee that you will consistently have the healthy food you want to eat available. When you're running low, it's time to go.

I've mentioned the *"when"* a few times already if you've been paying attention (also refer to #8 below, under "Keys to Successful Eating"). The most important when (and what) of your eating habits refers to your carb intake. Exercise (walking, hiking, playing tennis, running, biking, swimming, lifting weights, etc.) improves the insulin sensitivity of your cells making it easier for glucose (energy) in your blood to be taken up and used as energy by your cells, namely muscle cells, rather than floating around in your blood stream and being stored as glycogen or body fat later.

Those who don't exercise and/or have the unfortunate circumstance of prediabetes or type II diabetes usually have poor insulin sensitivity, and they're considered "insulin resistant". When they eat a lot of carbs and especially the refined kinds in baked goods, white bread, crackers, chips, etc., their blood glucose will increase. This in turn increases insulin secretion to attempt to shuttle the blood glucose into the cells and out of the blood. If the cells are insulin resistant, those cells won't be able to take up the glucose as efficiently and they will have the high blood sugar (or hyperglycemia) that is characteristic of type II diabetes victims that isn't quite as easily controlled like it is for a healthy individual.

Therefore, eating a majority of your carbs around exercise (and actually consistently exercising) is an important habit for maintaining or achieving a certain level of leanness and good carb tolerance. Pairing your carb snacks like fruit with fat, fiber and/or protein will help to slow the digestion down of those carbs as well as reduce the ensuing blood sugar and insulin spike, keeping your blood sugar – and energy levels – steady all day long. No need to get carried away with this either, the post-exercise effects on insulin sensitivity for most people likely won't last much longer than a day, so you're going to have to keep exercising to hold onto those benefits (17).

When it comes to eating around your workouts, *what* you consume and *when* you consume it is going to be partially dependent upon your own personal preference.

To give yourself a steady stream of energy, consuming a small snack or meal ~2 hours before a workout should give you plenty of time to digest part or most of that food and use it for energy. If you must eat immediately before your workout, the same applies but likely just in smaller portions so you don't end up with an upset stomach or feel sluggish from eating too much food. Your pre-and post-workout meals should mainly focus on carbs and protein, with limited or smaller amounts of fat. Fat slows the digestion of those carbs and protein delaying their digestion and use for energy during and after your workout. If you're eating a balanced meal post-training that includes plenty of protein and carbs, don't worry quite as much about eating "low-fat" as it's not going to make or break your progress.

To keep things simple, I advise (and personally prefer) clients and especially athletes to just eat your post-workout meal as soon as you can. The research on the "anabolic window" is sort of all over the place, so I live by "the sooner the better" when it comes to post-workout carb- and protein-centered nutrition for optimizing recovery (18).

One of the most popular questions ever pondered is whether eating carbs late at night is bad. If you want to trust another credible source's advice and it's different than mine, then I encourage you to follow that advice and *see* how your body responds to it.

The best way I can explain this to you is relating it to a car – which has been done by several other sources in one way or another – with your body being the car and gas being carbohydrates.

Let's say you have a gas tank that is half full and you fill it up on your way to work which is a daily two-hour commute. Your car is going to burn through some of that gas and you're going to be able to put more in later on without it spilling over.

Now, let's say you fill your car on the way to work just like you usually do, but you get a call from your sick kid that causes you to turn around and stay home and not use any of that gas. Later that evening, after no gas has been used because the car has been sitting in your garage all day, you decide to put more gas in the car (because your car craves it for fuel, of course). Since not driving your car had burned no gas, the gas inevitably spills over and makes a mess all over the place.

Your body could be like this car. If you burn the fuel you put in it (carbs being the preferred and quick energy source), eating carbs later in the day isn't going to "make you fat". It's much more so about the total amount of carbs and calories you're consuming each day.

If you exercise in the evening, before and after that workout can be a good time to eat the majority of carbs you consume in a day because your muscles are ready to use those carbs for good (like muscle growth, energy, recovery, and glycogen stores) instead of "spilling over" from an already-full tank, like eating a couple of high-carb meals and going overboard on calories overall on your rest day instead of on a high-intensity training day.

If you mindlessly snack on carbs late at night, it's likely not the *carbs* that would make you fat. It's more so how many *calories* you end up consuming as a result of those delicious salty or sweet snacks that provide hardly any nutrients or satiety. If you're worried about what to eat in the evening, try to focus instead on what you're eating that entire day and try to keep it as consistent as possible with regards to the amount and type of protein, fat and carbs you're consuming.

Where

Where you eat is going to have an impact on the quality, quantity and selection of food you consume. Eating and preparing your meals at home is almost always the best option because you can be certain what's going into the dish you're eating. When going out to eat, it *is* possible to treat yourself once in a while without feeling guilty and sabotaging your goals. Keep in mind, there are ways to treat yourself without going home feeling like crap and regretting it for the next 6 hours.

Solution

Restaurant Dining Tips

1. **Always order water** before any other beverage and make sure you *drink* it. This will obviously help with hydration and also help you feel fuller sooner. It can save you money and extra calories.
2. **Choose baked or broiled** over deep-fried or "crusted".
3. **Get vegetables steamed** instead of fried or covered in any mystery sauce.
4. **When ordering a sweet or baked potato,** don't feel the need to eat all of the butter, bacon bits, sour cream or brown sugar they provide for you; try asking for it on the side so you can decide how much you consume.
5. **Pasta dishes, especially alfredo, can be a nightmare for your**

waistline. These dishes are notorious for being extremely high in fat, carbs, calories, and sodium. If you're curious, just ask the restaurant for the nutrition facts before you order.

6. **Words like "crusted, smothered, glazed, or dipped"** are usually precursors to a very high sodium/fat/calorie recipe or sauce. Try to avoid them unless you know what that added crust/sauce/glaze is made from and are OK with it.

7. **Be picky.** Ask questions you want to know about preparation and don't be afraid to ask to substitute certain sides for healthier options or get a dish without its "signature" sauce on it. You can always ask for extra veggies instead of the side of chips, potatoes, or fries (and then mooch a few off your neighbor). You're a generous tipper anyways, right?

8. **Take some home.** Unless you're like me, the portions you get in a restaurant are likely larger than what you'd normally consume at home. Don't feel obligated to finish all of it. Most times you can probably get two meals out of one order. If you're OK with re-heating food, take the portion you don't finish home with you and have it tomorrow (meal-prep you didn't have to prep!).

When eating at home, keeping your meals at the dinner table (away from TV and other distractions) is a useful tool when beginning to eat more consciously. Eating right in front of a TV can take your mind off the food and leave you wanting more after what's in front of you is gone. Mindless eating and eating quickly can happen for several reasons, and watching TV at the same time is one of them.

One thing a lot of people struggle with is eating well while traveling or on vacation. You could, of course, just travel and follow my 10 tips ("Keys to Successful Eating") and see how well you can stick to them. Or, you could just do your best to make a conscious effort to eat mindfully at all (or at least most) meals and snacks. Believe me, I love to indulge on vacation like nobody's business. But I do it mindfully throughout the entire trip, and I make sure to get my exercise in, especially on days when I might hit a nice sushi buffet.

In my eyes, the most important things to consider while traveling or taking a vacation include planning (whether it's food you bring with or just where you're going to eat), packing snacks (that won't go bad), and drinking enough water.

While planning, consider checking restaurant menus ahead of time, eating a healthy meal before going out on a day trip or to any destination where the food choices are unknown, and knowing when and where you're going to eat that day so you don't end up famished at the exact moment you walk by a conjoined chilidog and ice cream stand. Planning transitions right into packing snacks.

Pack filling and nutritious snacks that last all day without going bad or getting crushed in a bag such as raw nuts, apples, carrots or protein bars. If you find yourself hungry in between meals or can't find a place to eat a decent meal, then you'll be prepared with something to hold you over. Not only that, but you'll save money by not buying usually over-priced goodies that are the norm on any vacation that won't provide you with very much nutrition or satiety.

Lastly, drinking enough water especially applies to traveling. It's so easy to forget to bring enough water when you're going to go on a walk around an area you've never seen before, go on a lengthy tour, or take a hike. By the end of a typical vacation day, you're likely going to be dehydrated if you don't plan ahead. I don't go anywhere without a water bottle and I even find this happening to me once in a while when traveling. If it happens to someone who is used to drinking about 200 ounces of water per day, my guess is you've had trouble with it too.

Why

Why is a biggie – why do you eat in the first place? Why did you choose Reese's Puffs for breakfast instead of oatmeal? Why do you eat vegetables every day? Why did you decide to get fast food for lunch? The number of questions you may ask yourself *"why"* you ate something can be endless and even frustrating.

The problem most people have is they just plain don't think about why they're choosing what they are. Whether they're going out to eat or eating a frozen dinner at home, there's no real health-driven reason behind it. To become *really* in tune with what you're eating and why you're eating it, you can think about what each food is going to do for your body, your goals, and your long-term health.

Health Tip to Try

Think about what that particular food you're choosing to eat is doing for your health. Does it mostly contain: protein, fiber, fat, healthy carbs, sugar, micronutrients? If you can be sure that it contains something your body needs or will benefit from, chow down; if not, reconsider and look at your options.

Solution

Look at *why* you eat and when you eat, beyond just what you might have filled into your dietary recall earlier. Asking yourself why you eat can be one of the simplest ways to open your eyes to the reasons you choose to eat certain foods at certain times.

For example, Sharon walks into the kitchen at 10pm and opens the freezer. She sees popsicles, ice cream, and ice cream sandwiches (the frozen fruits and veggies are invisible to the human eye at this time of night). She decides to dish up a large bowl of ice cream and adds chocolate syrup on top. She inhales it while watching a re-run of Seinfeld (because who can't resist Seinfeld and ice cream) and then scolds herself for eating that so late at night when she wasn't even hungry to begin with. Sharon could've approached this situation in three ways.

The first way, described above, has happened to me in the past multiple times and probably every person who enjoys some type of treat. She wanted something sweet, even before realizing why, what, and how much she was eating, and suddenly it was gone. The next day she vows to eat no junk food or ice cream and to exercise for an extra half hour to burn off last night's treat (good luck).

The second way she could've approached this was to just wait a minute, drink a glass of water, see if she still feels "hungry" enough for that ice cream, and after finally realizing she isn't hungry and doesn't need that right before bed, she skips the treat (good job, Sharon).

The third way (and my personal favorite) she could've approached the situation was to decide, *yes, I do want to taste some of that ice cream, but I don't want it to ruin my day – I've eaten really well today.* So she takes one spoonful of ice cream, puts the ice cream away, eats that *one* spoonful, and adds a small handful of fiber-full, heart-healthy, blood-sugar-stabilizing, protein- and fat-filled almonds to the snack to stave off hunger (brilliant!). She doesn't go crazy or feel deprived, and she makes a healthier snack out of the situation. It's a win-win!

Once you start becoming more conscious of your food choices each day, consider thinking about what you're eating and why before you eat it. It's quite simple: if you have a long workout that included 30-45 minutes of resistance training and you decided to run two miles afterwards, you might decide to eat a chicken breast (for <u>protein</u> and <u>muscle recovery</u>), half a cup of quinoa (for protein again, <u>fiber,</u> and a good source of <u>carbs</u> for <u>muscle recovery</u>) and a side of mixed veggies you sautéed in garlic, oregano, thyme and one tsp of olive oil (<u>micronutrients</u>). The underlined words all indicate a reason you may have chosen to eat that certain food and they were good, health-conscious reasons.

Now, for the layperson who decided to do that same workout and came home to eat a bowl of chips (not optimal carbs or a healthy fat, virtually no protein for needed recovery) and sausage pizza (not a lean source or very high in protein) for dinner, sure, they're getting some protein (from the sausage and cheese), carbs (refined flour), and fat (from the sausage and cheese). But, when looking at the meal described earlier that has everything you might need after a workout, the latter meal not only is lacking in the nutrient-dense foods you want, but it's likely going to leave you feeling sluggish and searching for more calories compared to the satiating first meal described.

When faced with a decision like this, all one has to do it ask themselves, what are these chips doing to aid my recovery from that workout? If you can't come up with a good answer, the answer is likely you should be choosing a different food.

Another example of conscious decision making would be choosing lunch on a workday. You ate a great breakfast at 7am of oats with almond butter, walnuts, flaxseed, and a banana. You're sitting at your desk from 8am-noon and have only gotten up once to use the restroom. You decide to order pasta from the Italian place across the street (of course, it comes with two garlic-butter breadsticks and a soda). You haven't exercised, you've hardly stood up or walked around all morning, you haven't burned off many of the carbs you've eaten for breakfast, and you decide to get a meal that is 85% carbs, 10% fat, and 5% protein. What this meal likely does after you eat it is spike your blood sugar (refined flour from the white pasta and breadsticks), load you up with probably a good 100+ grams of carbohydrates, and leave you crashing at 2:30pm, at which point you buy a soda from the vending machine as a pick-me-up. If you would've just asked yourself before ordering, *what is this meal doing for my body or my health goals*, it's more than possible that you could've decided on a better option for the middle of a low-activity workday. How about a salad with tuna, cottage cheese, and veggies on top? Stir-fry with grilled chicken and loads of veggies and a moderate portion of noodles? Both would be more than optimal workday lunches compared to the former.

If you try thinking about why you're choosing to eat what you eat at any given moment, you'll even start to learn a few things that you may not have noticed before – like how a certain food/meal makes you feel whether you eat it before or after exercising or in the middle of a sedentary day. You'll begin to learn what foods are higher in protein, carbs and fat and why those foods feel better for your body at certain times. Remember, your goal is to learn as much as you can about your own body throughout this process.

How

How to eat is not a hard question to answer – you take the food and place (or cram) it into your mouth. How to cook and be prepared each day, on the other hand, is a hard task to answer to.

Health Tip to Try

When eating a meal, don't watch TV, surf the Internet, or browse social media on your phone. Listen to music or just enjoy the food and/or company you're with. Doing something distracting while eating can take your mind off the task at hand – which should be fueling your body. This can lead to mindless eating, overeating, and not actually enjoying the food you have in front of you.

Solution

Cooking and planning can be as easy as one, two, three.

1. **Know what you're having for the next meal**
   a. I get laughed at, believe it or not, for asking what's planned for dinner while I'm eating lunch with someone. Joke's on them, because I'm just used to being prepared.
   b. If you know you want some type of frozen meat/fish for dinner, take it out of the freezer so it can thaw and reduce

the cooking time by half for the next meal. If you don't know what you want for dinner, now is the time to plan; if you need ingredients for the food you want, plan on when those ingredients are going to be picked up.

2. **Know how long it takes to prepare**

   a. If you don't take 10 seconds to think about how long it's going to take to prepare and eat your next meal, you could fall into the trap so many people fall into each day and end up running out of time and eating fast food on your way to your next activity. Take the time to think it through and you won't have to rush.

3. **Add in extras**

   a. By extras, I mean tasty, aromatic, health-boosting contents such as garlic and herbs and spices (you should definitely have in your kitchen... hint, hint) such as basil, oregano, thyme, rosemary, cumin, crushed pepper, turmeric, ground red pepper, cloves, etc. Some of these contents, although small, have been shown to have medicinal-like effects within the body you don't want to miss out on, not to mention they can make food taste and smell much more appealing.

   b. Extras might also include the healthy fats that can be used to cook your protein or veggies such as olive, sunflower, grapeseed or coconut oil, to name a few.

If you wonder why chicken and mixed vegetables with brown rice is boring to you but delicious to another person, ask them what they do when preparing it. It's amazing how many people have no idea how good a simple meal can taste when you have a full spice rack and different types of fats to sprinkle onto whatever you're preparing.

Here's one of my go-to favorite meals:

Chicken and Veggies (total preparation time: 15-20 minutes)

Start by putting your thawed chicken in a covered pan on the stove on medium to medium-high heat with 1 Tbsp. of coconut oil. Flip after ~5-8 minutes when the outside of the chicken is completely white. When it is close to being done (~5-8 more minutes), season it how you wish (lemon pepper is one of my favorites).

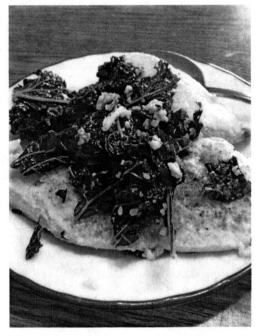

As the chicken is cooking, wash a sweet potato, poke holes in it with a fork and wrap it in a paper towel. Microwave it for 2.5-3 minutes, rotate it and cook again for 2.5-3 minutes.

As the sweet potato and chicken are cooking, place another pan on the stove on medium-high heat and fill it full of whatever veggies you'd like (one bag of frozen mixed veggies works great per two people, or for some leftovers) and 1 Tbsp. of fat.

Once the frozen veggies are just about done and the sweet potato is finished cooking, cut up the sweet potato and put it in the same pan as the veggies. Sprinkle on turmeric, oregano, basil, thyme, and minced garlic (fresh or from a jar) and let cook for the last 5-8 minutes, stirring occasionally.

If you have a very large pan, you can put all of these contents in the same pan in the following order: thawed chicken (cook on both sides until 75% done and then add next portion), frozen/fresh veggies (cook until 75% done and then add next portion) and lastly the microwaved and sliced sweet potato. Once everything is in the pan, season to your liking and let cook for ~5 more minutes, stirring occasionally until done.

Meal prepping on Sundays or another day that works for you is a great way to save time. You can bake 10 chicken breasts, boil/bake 6 sweet/regular potatoes, fry up or hard-boil 8 eggs, cook 4 cups of oats, and stir-fry 3 bags of frozen veggies in about an hour, separate them into containers you can take with you or store in your fridge, and be done with "cooking" for the entire week. If you don't like reheated foods and are a busy person, at least consider prepping your protein for the week because that is likely going to take the most time to cook compared to other things such as veggies or carbs that can be whipped up in 10 minutes or less. Even prepping two days at a time is going to save you a lot of time and will start you moving in the right direction.

If you don't already consume oats or eggs on a regular basis, I highly recommend giving each of my favorite recipes a try before you give up on these two versatile foods. I like to eat my oats cold (overnight oats) or just heated up in a microwave. If you prefer to cook them on the stove, then feel free to prepare them that way as well, but you'll be better off cooking for more than one day at a time to save time. And if you're still one of those who are afraid of the dietary cholesterol in egg yolk (which are packed with nutrients) and its effects on your cholesterol or heart disease risk, there's no need to worry anymore (19, 20). Here are a few of the different ways I prepare oats and eggs on a daily basis:

Chocolate Peanut Butter Banana Oats (3 minutes)

Pour one serving of 100% old-fashioned oats in a glass bowl and fill it with as much water/almond milk/etc. as you prefer for consistency. (I fill the bowl with water and let soak for ~5 minutes before microwaving to soften the oats.) Cut up half of a banana and place it with 5 dark chocolate chips on top of the oats, or replace the dark chocolate chips with 1/2 scoop of chocolate whey protein powder (and add the protein powder after microwaving). Microwave on high for ~1 minute. Take the bowl out and add an optional 1/2 tsp of unsweetened cocoa powder, 1 tsp of ground flaxseed, cinnamon to taste, the rest of the banana (if you prefer it) and 1 Tbsp. of natural peanut butter. Mix together and enjoy your "dessert" for breakfast.

Whey Protein Flavored Oats (3 minutes)

Pour one serving of 100% old-fashioned oats in a glass bowl and fill it with as much water/almond milk/etc. as you prefer for consistency (I fill the bowl with water and let soak for ~5 minutes before microwaving). Microwave on high for ~1 minute. Depending on the flavor of protein powder you have, that will help decide what extra add-ins you may want to choose. If you have chocolate flavored protein, try mixing it with 1 Tbsp. of almond/peanut butter and half a banana. If you have vanilla, try mixing it with just cinnamon and 1 Tbsp. of almond/peanut butter. If you have a fruit flavor such as strawberry, try mixing it with any other type of berry or a banana. Always consider adding a bit of ground flaxseed (once you know how much your body can handle at a time), 1 serving of chia seeds or ground nuts such as pecans or walnuts for a healthy fat.

This concept goes great with plain Greek yogurt as well. Mix ~1 scoop of whey protein with 1 serving (or smaller if you don't want to consume as many calories or can't handle the large portion) of plain Greek yogurt, stir it up and add in the extras you'd like, especially the healthy fat like I mentioned above. It's like ice cream for dessert, except minus the unnecessary sugar and extra calories, and plus much more protein, better gut health and added healthy fats.

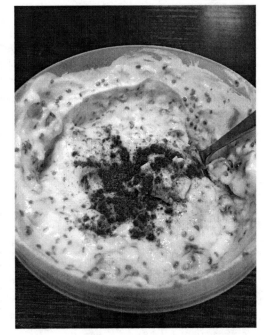

Overnight Oats (3 minutes)

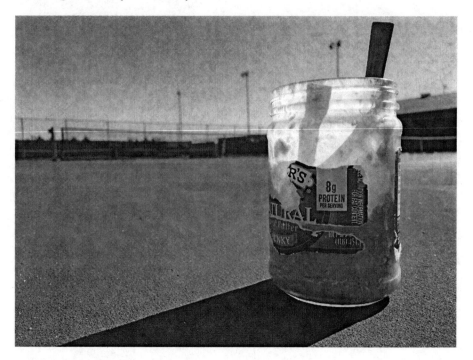

These are best made in a closeable container so they can be taken with you wherever you go when you don't have time to cook (hint, hint), and there are a lot of options when making overnight oats. Here's one:

Mix 1/2 cup of plain Greek yogurt with 1/2-1 scoop of your favorite protein powder. Add in 1/2-1 serving of plain oats and stir together (if you like a smoother texture, add in a little water or milk/almond milk). Add in a healthy fat such as flax seed, chia seed or some variety of ground nuts. Now add in the extra options I mentioned above such as peanut/almond butter, cinnamon, berries, etc. depending on the flavor you want to predominate your overnight oats. Store them in the fridge and consume them cold tomorrow.

Here's a second option:

Pour one serving of oats into a container/jar and fill it with the amount of liquid (water, almond milk, etc.) that you prefer. For flavor, add one or more of the following: almond/peanut butter, cinnamon, 1/2 scoop of your favorite protein powder, dried fruit, berries, unsweetened cocoa powder, banana, honey, etc. Then, of course, add in a healthy fat just like before. My favorite add-ins with my oats soaked in unsweetened almond milk or Fairlife chocolate milk are peanut butter, flaxseed, chia seed, cinnamon, chocolate protein powder (if I'm not using Fairlife milk) and a banana.

Eggs (10-15 minutes)

Scrambled eggs (or in a burrito for extra carbs) are great for two reasons. First, they're very quick and easy to make and they're hard to mess up unless you leave them on the stove for 15 minutes unattended. Second, you can pack 1-4 servings of different types of veggies (and always leafy greens) into one plate of scrambled eggs. It's really a win-win.

Option 1: Scrambled Eggs/Scrambled Egg Breakfast Burrito (10-15 minutes)

Heat up a pan and put in 1 Tbsp. of coconut or olive oil. Add in diced up veggies such as mushrooms, onions, bell peppers, leafy greens, etc. and let cook as long as you prefer. If you want the veggies crunchy, put the greens and eggs in right away; if you want them softer, then let them cook for ~5 minutes along with the greens you choose before you put the eggs in. After your veggies are cooked to your preference, add in 2-4 whole eggs. Sprinkle on some of your favorite herbs/spices (this should be done every time in my opinion) such as oregano, black pepper, ground cayenne pepper, basil, turmeric, thyme, rosemary, or cilantro, etc. and stir the eggs until done. Adding a little bit of meat or cheese would be done at this point if you want them as well. Heat up your tortilla (remember to check the fiber/protein content) for 15 seconds and put half of a sliced avocado on it and if you enjoy hummus, 1 Tbsp. of hummus on the tortilla as well. Pour on the eggs along with some optional salsa.

Option 2: Sunny-Side Up (~10 minutes)

Heat up a pan on low-medium heat along with 1 Tbsp. of coconut or olive oil. Put in your 2-4 whole eggs, attempting not to break the yolks. Cover the eggs with your favorite herbs and spices, a few minced veggies, and 1-2 handfuls of leafy greens and cover the pan. Optional add-ins to use include real cheese and/or a small amount of meat such as sliced turkey breast or leftover protein from your dinner the night before (salmon is great too). Once you can shake the pan and the egg yolks are done to your lik- 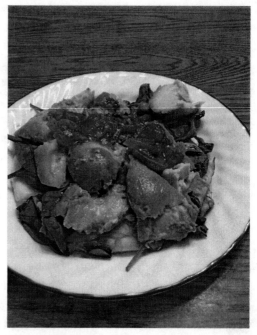 ing (~6-8 minutes) and the greens are wilted from the moisture, transfer your creation onto a plate and add avocado and salsa on top. I make this more than anything else when I'm in a hurry because it's the most convenient. It takes about 2 minutes to put everything in the pan, I can let it cook while I shower or eat my oats (as long as you know how long it takes to cook based on how hot you turn your stove on), and it's done when I come back to it.

Oats and eggs are extremely cheap, nutritious, filling and versatile. Experiment with your own favorite recipes until you have a collection of options that never get old.

Another "how" when it comes to eating has to do with how you feel. If you feel as if you have trouble digesting some types of food or don't feel satisfied until 10 minutes after you're done eating and it hits you like a sack of sweet potatoes, not chewing enough or drinking enough water before or during your meals might be your problem (along with eating too fast).

Chewing more not only slows down the eating process and allows you to feel satiated earlier, but it also helps you enjoy the food you're eating and works to help your stomach and digestive tract break down and digest that particular food more easily. If you stuff yourself quickly and immediately feel like laying down to unbutton your pants more than just on Thanksgiving, losing/maintaining weight is going to prove more difficult than it needs to be. For lasting control over your eating technique, strive to regularly eat slowly and *just* until you're satisfied and be able to stop at that point. This brings us to, "Keys to Successful Eating".

Keys to Successful Eating

These are 10 important key points to keep in mind about your diet that will help you stay on track long term and find healthy eating a whole lot easier. Remember, trying something for a few consecutive meals, days or weeks is what ultimately should determine if you continue that habit or not. If you feel good or "see" good (good results), keep it going. If you noticeably don't feel good, stop. If you're unsure if it makes you feel better or worse, give it more time until it's clear to you.

1. Drink more water
   a. At least 1/2 your body weight in pounds, in ounces per day. If you're an active person, that number probably needs to increase depending on how much you sweat. *Always* start your day by drinking a glass of water when you wake up, before you consume anything else (yes, even before coffee). It's the easiest way to start your day off on the right foot, even if you miss breakfast.
2. Aim for 90% "good" eating, and 10% "not so good" eating
   a. If you stick to a healthy diet (real foods - not sugary, processed, man-made products) most of the time, planning to treat yourself with a *controlled* portion of whatever you love won't feel like a bad thing, and it shouldn't.
   b. Another percentage point to think about consistently is not eating to "100% full". Precision Nutrition teaches this as a goal for *everyone* to reach when it comes to eating. Stopping at 80% full during each meal takes practice (and eating slowly), but it can yield great results and can be done anywhere, anytime.

3. Check yourself before you wreck yourself (reiterated)
   a. All this means is to ask yourself before you eat something – what is this doing for my body? Is it helping my health or hurting my health?
4. Treat yourself regularly
   a. This could mean a serving of dark chocolate every day, a spoonful of ice cream, or eating a meal not usually on your diet plan once or twice a week (not a massive Thanksgiving-style buffet...). The best way to stay on track and have a treat not turn into a disaster is to *plan* it into your regular diet.
5. Don't look for foods with health claims
   a. If the food claims to be healthy, showing a nice big label with a star on it, chances are it isn't. Stick to real foods that don't have a paragraph of ingredients or foods that don't have a nutrition label at all, like produce and fresh fish and meat.
5.5. When in doubt, read it out. If the label reads these ingredients anywhere, try to limit your intake on a regular basis
   b. If the label has sugar or a disguised name for sugar (molasses, high fructose corn syrup, anything ending in "ose") in the first 3 ingredients, try not to buy it regularly. This applies if the ingredients list is a paragraph of things you can't pronounce (exception: some "_____extracts" that may be in an immune-boosting or gut-healing supplement or probiotic, those can be tough to pronounce no matter what).
   c. Hydrogenated or partially-hydrogenated oils = trans fats. Even if trans fat is listed as "0g per serving", these foods still contain trans fats (less than 0.5g per serving can still add up). If there is one food or type of foodstuffs we're currently confident is detrimental/offers no benefit to our health, it's trans fats.
   d. There are certainly other things on labels – like artificial colors, flavors, and preservatives – that would be beneficial to limit as well. I just find that the two above examples are most often found in the most common processed (and fairly addicting) snack foods and meals.

6. Grocery shop mostly on the outside of the store
   a. This is where the "whole foods" you hear about are located. Aside from most beans, nut butters, oils, oats, herbs, spices and some others, the stuff on the inside of the store isn't food; it's a processed food-product. If you wonder why all the packaged/processed foods are on the inside, think about how inconvenient it would be to have the food-stockers need to wheel the fresh meat, fish, eggs, dairy, etc. through all the isles of the store every day. Processed foods can sit on the shelf for a long time without needing daily re-stocking, and that's why they're in the middle of the store.
7. Plan your meals
   a. It doesn't have to be prepared a week in advance, but if you have no idea what you're eating for lunch that day the chances of you eating something you might regret are pretty high. This is one of the most important keys to staying on track with a healthy diet.
8. Eat your carbs at the right time
   a. Focus your high-carb meals/snacks before or after your workouts and if you're consuming just carbs for a snack/meal, add a protein and/or fat to it as well. The goals here are to use those pre- or post-workout carbs for quickly-usable energy and to keep your blood sugar as stable as possible between your snacks and meals to keep you from crashing and craving more carb-rich foods (which usually end up being junk food). Consume simple carbs such as fruit juices, soda, sweets, crackers, etc. mainly pre- and post-workout. This timing may also be more important for athletes or those who compete in any type of prolonged athletic or exercise event that may deplete muscle glycogen (think of a weekend-long volleyball or tennis tournament or having two running races on back-to-back days, when replenishing your muscle and liver glycogen becomes more important between athletic events to restore as much energy for the next event as possible).
      i. This "key" is also dependent upon the person. If you eat a carb-rich meal and feel like a slug that needs a

nap 1-2 hours later, there's a good chance you don't tolerate carbs as well as your buddy who has no problem eating that meal and feeling good. If you feel fantastic having high-carb meals or snacks and you never notice a crash in energy shortly after eating, then you're more likely to be able to follow this key a little more loosely (chances are you're generally leaner than your heavy-set buddy if that's the case as well).

9. Consume protein with every meal
    a. This not only goes for every meal, but also, when possible, every snack as well – and it's not just for super-active athletes. It takes more energy from your body to digest protein than it does to digest carbs, making a small impact on how many calories your body burns at rest every day. Protein is vital for your well-being and is very satiating. It's key to recovery and a lean and strong body.

10. Eat your veggies
    a. If you don't consume much fruit, set your ideal veggie intake at a minimum of 2-3 servings per day, with a serving being the size of your fist. If you eat a lot of fruit each day, a general rule to consider is to consume at least an equal number of servings of vegetables to fruits. If you insist on having 5 servings of fruit in a day, aim for 5 or more servings of vegetables that day as well. Plants that vary in color like different leafy greens, broccoli, asparagus, mushrooms, beets, bell peppers, cherry tomatoes and red onions are great examples. Fiber, micronutrients and color from vegetables (and fruits) should be a daily part of your meal plan. (There isn't a scientific reason for this rule of eating equal or greater veggies than fruits – it's just a basic way to think about consuming enough veggies each day when fruits tend to be easier to eat and tastier to most people, sometimes leaving veggies by the wayside – which are usually lower in calories but still offer great benefits.)

Keys to Your Kitchen

There are many ways to organize your kitchen and make it more conducive to reaching your goals. These are a few things you can do to keep yourself on track with your eating goals, your preparation goals, and your ability to save money at the grocery store.

1. **Keep your healthiest go-to's where you can see them first.** That means your fruits, veggies, lean proteins, healthy snacks, beans, etc. When you're really hungry or don't have a plan of what to eat, you'll likely grab the first thing you see (this is also one of the main reasons why meal prepping is so helpful).

2. **Keep it clean.** Your dishes (as often as possible), your stove, your microwave, your countertop; nothing makes lazy people want to go out to eat quicker than looking at a nasty 4-day-old meatball stain on a white countertop. The cleaner it is, the more likely you are to want to use it the right way – by cooking.

3. **Know where everything is.** Keep certain types of foods or food groups in the same area of the fridge, freezer and cupboard so you know where to find them – like when you're looking for a complex carb to make with dinner or some type of fresh vegetable to cook with your steak.

4. **Don't forget about your produce.** (Remember #1 also.) It's extremely easy to buy plenty of fresh fruits and veggies for the week, accidentally hide them behind leftover lasagna in the back of the fridge, and then discover them two weeks later wilted, moldy and seemingly growing into a different species. "Buying healthy food is so expensive" *they* say; *they're* right, especially when *they* don't actually eat the produce they bought for $2.99/lb.

5. **Stock your freezer.** The best thing about stocking your freezer with healthy options such as lean meats, fish, a variety of vegetables, and berries is if and *when* you run out of fresh healthy options in your fridge/pantry, you will always have a backup plan. Take things out of your freezer when you need them and remember how much of your favorite foods you have left so you can re-stock next time you go shopping. When go-to items like beans, frozen salmon, chicken, veggies, etc. are on sale, stock up to save money in the long run.

6. **Invest in a spice rack.** Herbs and spices are what separate the bland cook from the person who loves eating the same thing week after week. Not only will your food taste and smell better/different each time you prepare it with different combinations, but you'll be getting a plethora of phytochemicals from the plants that herbs and spices come from that will add to the vibrant life you're trying to live. Don't forget about pre-minced garlic if you go that route either, which is usually stored in the fridge, not the spice rack.

Where to Adjust Your Diet

Re-visit your food log, or simply fill in from memory the following table concerning the foods you consider "good" and "bad" in your regular diet and why you consider them as such. If you haven't filled out the food log, just fill in the table with common foods you eat.

The Good, the Bad, and the Ugly

Good Food	Why	Bad Food	Why
Oats	Good carbs, fiber, protein, whole food, easy b-fast	Diet soda	Artificial, chemicals, makes me crave more
Salmon	Healthy fat, protein, versatile leftovers	Potato chips	High calorie, easy to overeat, nutrient-void

Table 2.8

I hope looking at this table can give you an idea of how "good" or "bad" your diet is in your own eyes so far. The good news is – it's simple to make changes (I didn't say easy).

How to Adjust Your Eating Habits

When deciding where to adjust your diet, first look at the areas of "bad" food/drink that stand out to you the most. Start with the worst areas that are clearly holding you back, and move up to the less harmful – but still needing improvement – types of foods afterward.

For example, let's say there are two foods or drinks that you eat every day or every other day that you know aren't good for your health. One of them you're pretty confident you can either cut out of your diet, find a better substitute for, or just plain reduce the amount you consume. The other, you CANNOT live without and have no idea how you're going to conquer that fear (you just got cold sweats even thinking about not eating that food/consuming that drink).

The smarter choice to adjust first would clearly be the food/drink you're pretty confident you can make adjustments to, even if it's the "less bad" of the two. This will help you not only get a good start on improving the weak areas in your diet, but it will give you confidence in knowing you *can* adjust areas of your diet without losing your mind. Then you can move onto the next challenge.

When changing certain eating habits, start small. Small adjustments are the best and easiest ways to improve your health long term. When completely cutting out a food or beverage you currently consume daily or multiple times a day, withdrawal symptoms can occur and most certainly send you crawling back to that item. We don't want a yo-yo diet; we want slow and steady improvements over time, even if those improvements require some "up and down" along the way.

Let's say you drink two cans of diet soda per day and you know you shouldn't because you always want a certain junk food after and it's costing you a lot of money in soda and snacks. A great way to start attacking this habit is by just reducing that number to one can per day while replacing the other can with a glass of water (or another less-harmful beverage like flavored water to get you closer to the real thing) and see how you feel after about a week. No headaches, shaky hands, trouble focusing, or trouble sleeping? Great, next you can try reducing the amount a bit more – say to one can every other day. Still feel great a week or even two weeks later? Reduce it to two or three per week, and so on and so forth until consuming that drink occurs more so on special occasions. This is the safest and most effective way to change a negative habit.

What if you change the habit too quickly and start feeling withdrawal symptoms coming on or you find yourself craving that food/beverage? Easy, just go back to where you could maintain the adjustment you made and make the adjustment even smaller than you did the first time and test it for a longer period of time, like two or three weeks instead of just one.

Letting your body and mind adapt to what you're changing before you move onto bigger and better changes is vital at this point. The last thing you want is to feel deprived for a week and end up binging on that food or beverage because you just can't take it anymore. This is setting yourself up for failure (and a main reason why most *diets* fail). *Always make the smallest changes possible while still being able to make forward progress.*

The easier the habit change, the more likely you are to make that change and keep it long term, leading to more successful habit changes in the future. Even if you're thinking to yourself, *I'm hardly changing anything, there's no way this is going to help me lose 15lbs,* you're doing the right thing. You *are* changing something that will lead to more changes later on. You're learning about the process. Small progress *is* still progress.

Once you start working on changing the habits around the "bad" foods and are finding success, just keep attacking them slowly but surely. Don't be surprised if it takes you one or two months to reduce or eliminate even *one* of the "bad" foods on your list. If it takes that long but it ends up being permanent, then mission accomplished. To summarize, the process goes like this:

1. Choose *one* eating/drinking habit that is going to be improved
2. Reduce the amount you consume (or add an amount of a good food) by an amount you're confident you can handle every day
3. Keep that amount consistent every day for one to two weeks
4. If you fail with the habit, revert back to #2 and make the amount adjusted *smaller*
5. If you succeed with the habit, keep going for 2-4 more weeks with it (and increase the amount adjusted by a small margin if it's going well) until it becomes an easily-maintainable habit

6. Once you conquer that eating or drinking habit and are still moving forward, look at your list of "to-do's" and choose the next one

At the same time, don't forget to give yourself credit for the "good" foods in your diet you currently consume. Even if you drink a liter of soda a day, give yourself some credit for getting two servings of vegetables and two servings of lean protein each day too (and to remind yourself you're not failing). Positive reinforcement and positive self-talk will go a long way in helping you improve your eating habits. Food/eating is something we can think about multiple times per hour, per day. That is a lot of opportunity to either help your mental progress or hurt it.

Your goal regarding the "good" foods is now to increase them just as slowly as decreasing the "bad" until you're at the recommended amount or ideal amount for your body and activity level – and you *feel* better on a consistent basis. Work up to getting a few servings of healthy fats each day, several servings of fruits and vegetables, consistent amounts of quality protein at each meal and snack, and drinking enough water. Use as many of the other tools I've already gone over to assist you in the process, or any other tools that you have that may be more effective.

Influences on Your Diet

Look at the positive and negative influences on your diet and eating habits. Fill out the table below so you can examine what's helping you and what's hurting you.

Influences on Your Diet

Positive Influence	Why	Negative Influence	Why
I have a gym buddy	He/she keeps me on track	My co-workers	Always ask me to lunch at fast food joint
I get a discount in the cafeteria that has a great salad bar	Healthy options for protein, fat and veggies, and has variety every day	The dollar menu is right across the street	It's cheap, fast, and convenient

Table 2.9

Now, for my first example, the positive influence of a gym buddy can be very motivating for your health and fitness goals. This person probably pushes you to do better in the gym and talks about healthy eating when you're together as well.

The negative influence of coworkers consistently asking you to lunch at a fast food place can become a form of peer pressure. Those are the types of people who might know you don't want to eat that kind of food because you have specific health goals, but they ask regardless and might even banter you each time you turn them down. If you have a negative influence like that in your life, the best thing to do is remind them why you're choosing to eat what you are and that sometime you *will* come out with them and treat yourself, just not today (even if you don't intend to in the near future). Letting go of negative influences is a powerful skill to have and it will help you in other aspects of your life as well.

The simple goal for this part of the strategy is to consider how you could increase the number of positive influences you have and decrease the number of negative influences you have. Find a group to meet with – a class at your gym maybe. Think of anyone or anything that will help keep you accountable and add it to your list of positive influences.

Once you've dealt with a specific negative influence and it's no longer a problem for you, feel free to cross it off the table or put a check mark next to the box. The more negative influences you can conquer and the more positive influences you can reinforce and add, the easier it will be to maintain your healthier lifestyle, and maybe even positively influence those around you. Fill out this table, and over time work towards *doubling* the number of positive influences as negative influences.

Feel free to fill out a table similar to this for the other strategies in this book as well. Exercise, diet, stress, outlook, motivation, and lifestyle habits will all certainly have positive and negative influences impacting their success. The more positive and the less negative influences regarding any of these aspects you have in your life, the better off you're going to be – and you won't feel like you're at it alone.

Many studies have shown that social support is beneficial when it comes to physical activity across different age groups (21-23). Even though we're talking about diet at the moment, these two challenges go hand-in-hand. Those who struggle with staying active usually have trouble eating a healthy and balanced diet, and vice versa.

When you have a friend or family member, or several of them, by your side to support you along the way or at least to be a listening ear, there's a good chance you'll be more successful in your endeavors. Do your best to find like-minded people or groups that have common goals so you can bounce ideas off them, ask them for guidance, or even share some of what you've learned with them and be a helping hand to someone else as well.

Susan is your classic example of a busy mom. She has 15-20 pounds of extra weight she wants to lose and has wanted to lose for the past 10+ years. Just like most others, life got in the way. She has a desk job that keeps her seated most of her week and a dog that keeps her walking before and after work each day. Her eating habits aren't perfect while trying to please her kids (who can relate, right?) and she's tried multiple different strategies and different diets to lose weight.

I've watched her try different things with her diet and exercise and nothing ever seems to stick or prove worth the hassle. Finally, I got her to commit to trying to cut out *added* sugar just for one week to see how her body felt. Sure, she's tried "cutting back" before, but it has never been cut and dry to the point where you read a label, if it has any sugar or disguised name for sugar in it, you don't eat it no matter what. She also increased the amount of fruits, veggies, nuts, seeds and protein she ate each day as a result of the lack of processed food.

By the end of the first week, she had lost 4 lbs. More to her surprise, she felt great. She wasn't dreaming about the late-night ice cream or kettle corn. She wasn't hungry and she didn't feel deprived. The second week, she lost another 3 lbs and still felt like she could continue, so she did. What she discovered most importantly was after several days without added sugar and less processed foods, she felt more in-tune with her body's natural ability to tell itself when it's hungry and when it isn't.

This is the most important lesson from ditching the processed food – not that going cold-turkey can work or that she lost a few pounds and it was all the sugar's fault (it wasn't, she just ended up replacing those foods with more nutrient-dense foods) – but when you aren't feeding your body sugar and processed carbs regularly and you feed it what it needs – the right kinds of macros, plenty of micronutrients, and water – chances are you won't crave those processed foods like you used to. The feeling is different for everyone, just don't give up before the cravings reduce! (She currently eats some foods with added sugar in them each week but has improved while slowly changing those eating habits and she's maintaining quite well.)

Everyone sees the statistics on how much sugar Americans eat each day/year and they know it's bad and they know it needs to change. The problem is they don't know how to commit to it and see how their body will react. All it takes is reading a label. After one week, you could notice a difference in the way you feel throughout the day and the way you feel before and after eating each snack and meal. I'm also not telling you to never eat sugar again (because we both know that's not going to happen); just to see how your body feels and reacts to consuming *less* sugar from processed foods.

Stress

"Don't find fault, find a remedy; anybody can complain."

-Henry Ford

Where to Begin

I frequently ask others, and myself, "What is stress? Why are you stressed? What makes you stressed?" I can't really feel it inside me, I don't sense it in my actions (outside of good stress related to sports), but I hear others complaining about it daily.

Of course, there are different kinds of stress. Stress that is "good" may improve your mental clarity, your athletic performance or your quick decision-making skills. "Bad" stress may ruin your mood for the rest of the day, make you crave certain (usually unhealthy) foods or make it impossible to focus on routine daily tasks. Some people just cringe at the sound of the word, like many people at the sound of the word "moist". Stress is normal, but when out of control, can sometimes force a person into a downward spiral.

Stress has been shown to have negative consequences on weight, body composition, mood, eating habits, metabolic disease, immunity and relationships (1-8). The good kinds of stress – like those butterflies you get before getting pumped up for a race – and bad kinds – like wanting to pull your hair out over someone's annoying habit of chewing loudly – define your daily stressors.

Stress is a tricky subject. It can vary from person to person an immense amount and everyone's triggers are and can be very different as well. The following common sources of stress are just the beginning, but look at them and reflect on your own sources of stress and see how many of these you deal with.

1. Job
2. Family
3. Friends
4. Significant other
5. Money
6. Health
7. School
8. Change
9. Pressure to succeed
10. Driving
11. Social gatherings
12. Time
13. Planning events
14. Holidays

If you deal with some of these sources of stress on a daily or weekly basis, keep them in mind while reading the rest of this strategy. Try to play through some of your own stressful situations while reading my own examples and attempt to resolve them yourself. In this case, practice makes (near) perfect.

How I Manage Stressful Situations

To be able to manage stressful situations without letting them get to you seems like a gift. "Letting it go" and "brushing it off" can be extremely difficult at times, but with practice they can become automatic. Some of you are already reading this thinking, *pfff... he doesn't know me or my problems, who does he think he is?*

Maybe I'm an empty shell on the inside who doesn't really *care*, or maybe I've just figured out how to control my mindset when dealing with situations that would normally stress someone out. I'm going to give you a few examples of thinking through a stressful situation that *works*.

Stressful Situation #1

You have a school/work project (which requires Internet) deadline in an hour and your Internet connection just went out.

1. What are your options with the resources you currently have?
    a. Check your computer's Internet connection/Wi-Fi signal. Did it just disconnect, do you need to re-enter the password, do you need to disconnect and connect again?
    b. Restart your computer.
    c. Can you call your boss/professor/teacher and explain the situation to come up with a solution or extend the deadline?
    d. Can you find a different computer?
    e. Can you go to another location (coffee shop) with Wi-Fi?
    f. Do you really need an Internet connection to submit it off your computer, or will a smart phone work?
    g. Say screw it and go lift weights.
2. What's option A?
    a. Go with it, if it doesn't seem to work, go with option B.
    b. If option B fails, move on down the list, Santa Clause, because there *has* to be another solution.
3. Are any of the solutions working or getting you closer to fixing the problem?
    a. If not, and all viable options have busted then all you can do is wait it out, no need to stress now because you've thought through every possible situation to solve the problem and none of them worked – mainly – *you did the best you could with the resources you had.*
    b. Once in this situation, ask yourself what stressing out will do to positively impact the situation (if it won't positively impact it, which it usually doesn't, then think of what might positively impact it, like moving on, getting your mind off of it, talking to someone about the situation/asking for outside help, etc.).
    c. Once you can contact your boss/coworker/professor/ teacher, explain the situation and explain what you did (calmly) to try to fix the problem. Often times, you'll see that you can calmly talk about a stressful situation that

they could've avoided reacting in a negative way altogether. Do your best to think *before* you speak and think *before* you react.

b. Try to fight the urge to react how you normally would – if that normal reaction is one you don't desire. Remember how you felt and how your mood changed the last time this situation occurred.

2. The key is to remember that you *can* control how you respond to things, but you *can't* control how much of a doofus someone else is. Let your maturity and composure show through your actions.

3. Pity the other person.

a. Believe it or not, at times when I was losing a tennis match I probably should've won in college (frustrating and scary to think about, I know), one of the ways I stayed level-headed and didn't lose my cool was to remind myself of how happy I was with my performance, effort, sportsmanship, or another aspect of my life or personality that I evaluated as being "better" than my opponent's or just "good" in my own eyes. I would look at my opponent (whether I knew their personal life or not, but sometimes you could see their personality by how they played and interacted with you) and tell myself, "*I have better sportsmanship than them, I'm stronger than they are, I'm happier than they are*" and it would just simply make me feel better about a negative situation – losing to someone I can beat (and often make me play better too). When the outcome of something (the tennis match, because you can't control how well your opponent plays no matter how well you're playing) is out of your control, you can't let it control you.

b. When dealing with a difficult customer, co-worker, boss, or acquaintance, simply try to put yourself in their shoes and understand why they're acting the way they are. Maybe they have a rough personal life that's causing them to act a certain way that you wouldn't understand. Maybe the way their parents raised them to cooperate with others wasn't as great as the way your parents raised you to. There could be multiple reasons why someone acts in a somewhat unfitting way. Not letting their mood rub off on yours is the simple way to keep them from getting under your skin and affecting your mood the rest of the day.

4.   Smile
   a.   Even if the person you're dealing with has been a world-class a-hole, let your last words with them be accompanied by a smile. It's like losing a match to someone in tennis who had terrible sportsmanship, whined about your line calls, and tried to call a judge over for your apparent foot-faults. You know deep down your sportsmanship on the court is far better than his (making you a more enjoyable opponent to compete against) and you will get much further in life with that positive attitude you take with you off the court than he will. You shake hands, smile and say, *"great match, good luck in your next one"* and walk away. The smart people who may have a bad attitude will notice that. They might walk away thinking, *wow, that person has an amazing attitude even after losing* (I've walked away thinking this multiple times when playing kind opponents). Maybe they'll get lucky and some of your great attitude will even rub off on them.

These are three examples of ways to deal with fairly common problems. I'm sure you've heard of other techniques such as closing your eyes and counting to 10 or taking 5 deep belly breaths, which can both be beneficial as well.

Health Tip to Try

If something is about to tick you off or send you over the stressful edge, try looking at yourself from someone else's perspective and asking yourself, is this really worth ruining my mood over? Is what I'm freaking out about really THAT big of a deal in the grand scheme of things? We're literally flying through space on a tiny marble and I'm complaining about this? Word it how you wish, but seeing things from a different view can work wonders.

I don't recall where I heard the following statement, but it applies very well to this subject: "If you're stressed out about something, you're failing to see the bigger picture." Obviously, this isn't going to apply to everyone 100% of the time, but trying to stay positive is what's most important. Whatever works for you, use it to the best of your ability. As we'll get into different ways to motivate oneself, it's good to have more than one way to manage your stress as well.

Procrastination almost always leads to unwanted stress. If you have a stress problem, see if you have a procrastination problem. If you have a procrastination problem, see if it's due to a time management problem. If you stress about the future, then remind yourself that worrying about problems that haven't even presented themselves yet (and may *not* even present themselves) could be a main source of your preventable stress in other aspects of your life as well. Getting to the root causes of your stress is going to be the most important step in figuring out how to prevent it from occurring or reducing its impact.

You're stressing out about stressing out because you're stressed out. It happens to (almost) everyone. Remember past situations and learn from your mistakes so when the next opportunity to conquer stress appears you're well prepared. Attempt to live by these few principles and you too may be able to be as cool as a cucumber.

1. Accept the things you cannot change. "Easier said than done," I always hear. Well, once you've "done" it enough, it will become an easy habit. Plus, we won't have to hear that excuse anymore and then everyone wins.

2. Look for, and see, the silver lining. I do catch myself once in a while not doing this, but lucky for me I can notice it, change it, and get back on the right track. You can find a silver lining in just about every single situation; you just have to look for it. To avoid completely killing your ability to do this before you give it a try, avoid thinking you or anyone else is "downplaying" your problems or struggles. All that thought process is doing is justifying the way you're [negatively] reacting to it in your own mind. (Grieving over the loss of a pet or loved one doesn't really apply here, no need to get carried away.) You can't control what happens to you, but you can control how you react to it.

3. Do your best, don't stress, and forget the rest. If you've actually done your best – thought through every scenario, tried to solve the problem in front of you, gave it everything you've got –

then what do you have to worry about? Something I periodi-cally tell my athletes (whether you think it's wise or not) is that "you can't win 'em all". Which is very true in sports and in life. All you really can do is use the tools you have to try to accomplish your goals, work as hard as you can, and hope for the best possible outcome.

Caroline had a stress problem. She let people around her and events that happened to her get under her skin and affect her mood and attitude. You can probably relate to this because it's almost a daily occurrence for many people. Her stress would get to her and it would distract her from actually trying to solve the problem that was causing the stress in the first place.

I tried to help her with her stressful way of dealing with problems by first talking through them, much like I outlined in this strategy. My goal was to get her to step back, look at the situation, and think about the possible solutions to the problem without letting a quick emotional reaction get in the way of thinking logically (I know, this might be a stretch). If there were no solutions and she had done everything in her control, then there was nothing left to worry about. This was the hardest part because Caroline didn't like to feel like she had no control over a situation – but that's where most of her stress came from. Situations in which you have no control over or situations in which you don't know what the outcome will be can cause a lot of stress.

Getting Caroline to let go of her fixation on an outcome and just focus on what she *could* control (the process) was a helpful tactic for her with more practice. It didn't happen successfully the first, second, or even fifth time she tried to let go, but eventually it started to make more sense. She was able to focus on things in her control and feel blessed with what she did have control over.

When you're able to keep reminding yourself of what you're thankful for or happy about in your life (like, every single day) you will ditch more of the stress and negativity that comes along with that worrying. Take a deep breath and ask yourself if you can solve this problem. If you *can't* control it, then it *shouldn't* control you.

Outlook

"When everything seems to be going against you, remember that the airplane takes off against the wind, not with it..."

-Henry Ford

Where to Begin

An individual's outlook on life can vary from year to year, month to month, or day to day. Events can occur that inevitably change a person's mood; whether they're okay with it or not. I truly believe the happiest people on earth are the ones who have the right outlook and make the best out of each and every situation they encounter. The challenge is always *how* can we possibly keep the right outlook on a situation that seems less than fortunate. Remember, you can't control what happens to you, but you can control how you respond to it.

Have you ever experienced something that *should* be emotionally minuscule that turns out to be more than it should or a chain of events that makes you so mad and upset that it ruins your mood for the rest of the day? It happens to people all the time. You open up social media and see nothing but complaints of "first world problems" that are just ridiculous. "My new Lexus has a flat tire!! *insert crying emoji here* Why is life so unfair??" or "Just dropped my ice cream cone on the ground #dayruined". These people may just be venting, but in my opinion, deep down they probably have some major outlook issues, are consistently stressed, tend to complain about small details, and fail to see the bigger picture as opposed to being the type who can laugh at themselves in unfortunate situations.

A great example of this begins with me having a delicious snack (the details need not be fabricated). I was quite hungry and had over an hour until my dinner was ready, so I decided to have some muenster cheese wrapped in deli turkey. The first bite was so damn delicious (I don't eat that type of cheese or meat very often) and exciting I couldn't help but bite down hard on my tongue.

It was that kind of bite you know is going to bleed, swell and give you a slur for the next three days because you can hear a crunch inside both your ears as you chomp down. As I writhed in pain, I considered spitting the delicious but bloody food out of my mouth.

Being the champ that I strive to be, I kept chewing as I hopped around wincing from the pain in my tongue as to not waist the food, I hopped so far I stepped on the zipper of a jacket that was laying on the hardwood floor. (If you've ever done this or stepped on a Lego barefoot, you feel my pain.)

I then hobbled and hopped my way to the bathroom as I laughed at my pathetic self and I hit the elbow that was holding my mouth on the doorframe trying to make a tight right turn to check out my tongue. After another sad chuckle, a few deep breaths and some serious pity, I was over the sad series of events that just transpired and found it humorous that something like that could even happen to someone who considers himself pretty coordinated. Yes, my tongue was swollen and painful for the next few days and it made tasting food difficult, but the series of events was funnier, in my eyes, than it was frustrating.

Positivity

Starting off your day with a positive mindset might look like this: you wake up thinking, "Today is going to be a good day." You *get* to eat breakfast because you can afford it. You *have* a car, bike, or some type of transportation to get you to where you're going – work, errands, etc. You *can* communicate with those around you – co-workers, family, friends, the grocery store clerk – and you *can* make an impact on their day in a positive way. You *can* exercise after work because you're blessed with a normally functioning body. Lastly, you *get* to come home to dinner and/or your family for the rest of the evening. Sounds like a pretty boring day, doesn't it?

For someone with the wrong mindset, it can be. When comparing this to less-fortunate people living in the same area as you or people on the other side of the country or world, this day might seem like it's full of luxury. From someone else's standpoint, they might look at this lifestyle and be amazed you have a bedroom for each of your 3 kids, have a car, or have money to go out for dinner. Keeping a positive mindset for you at this point looks pretty easy.

It amazes me that people can have much more (relationship, career, money, possessions, etc.) than those close to them and still be less grateful. I like to think about this quote I can't take credit for: "The same water that hardens the egg softens the potato – it's not the circumstances, it's what you're made of." If you've never heard that before, go back and read it again, it's quite true.

Our circumstances shape how we act and who we become – if you haven't thought about that before, think back to your childhood or young adult years about an event or person who made a profound impact on how you act, what you value, or what you prioritize today. Often, we don't realize what makes the biggest impact on our lives until years later.

Negativity

Starting your day off with a negative mindset might look like this: you wake up getting an hour less sleep than you normally do, and think great, better get the coffee started so I can trudge through this day without smacking someone. You spill your bowl of oatmeal on the floor and don't have time to make and eat another one, so you walk out the door without grabbing any other food (which you did have available) thinking this day can only go up from here. You hit some traffic on the way to work, which just adds to the stress you started the day with. Your boss assigns you an extra project on top of your current workload, and now you're even more stressed than you were this morning, wondering when you're ever going to catch a break. You drive home after work and get pulled over for speeding away from the crappy day of work you just went through, and get a warning. *Awesome, the cherry on top of a perfect day.* You get home and inhale a pint of ice cream and sob to an episode of Grey's Anatomy because this day just didn't go your way.

Negativity adds to stress, and stress adds to negativity. They feed off of one another. Look back at my two examples above. If we compared a person with a positive mindset to someone with a negative mindset, the individual with the negative mindset would almost always have a higher level of stress and lower level of happiness day-to-day than the positive individual.

Your mindset, or outlook, as you go through your day will make all the difference in the world. Like any other habit or behavior change, this is going to take some getting used to, some trial and error, and most importantly, likely many, many failures before you feel "successful".

"It Could Be Worse"

Seeing the silver lining was something I used to struggle with. Like anything else, the more you practice, the better you become. I played tennis in college after a fairly easy high school tennis career. At times when I was younger, I would get pretty heated, like most tennis players, and let emotions get the best of me. Right around my sophomore and junior year of college, I changed drastically. I rarely got angry even during some of the most unfortunate times and my performance skyrocketed. How did I do it? To put it bluntly, I "stopped" caring about outcomes so much, and it carried over to my mindset outside of tennis as well. After all, tennis *is* just a game – but a game that can teach valuable lessons. What led to my change in mindset was mainly influenced by two events.

The first event occurred the summer after my sophomore year. I was a camp counselor and tennis instructor at Tennis and Life Camp at Gustavus Adolphus College in St. Peter, Minnesota. This place is a magical experience I would encourage anyone – 11 years old to 70 years old, experienced or beginner – to go to. The atmosphere is electric, loving, and encouraging. Having fun is easy, and creating meaningful and lasting relationships with campers of all ages is very common; even whilst seeing them for three short days. As the title says, it's Tennis *and* Life Camp. What I learned from my fellow instructors and the people who came to camp from age ~11 to 70 years would stay with me for a long time.

This camp opened my eyes to how lucky I am, and how lucky those individuals who came to camp were, to be playing this game. A tennis match can be an emotional roller coaster unlike any other sport. Having a positive mindset during the game of tennis at times can seem almost as difficult as taking a set off Roger Federer.

I had the privilege to meet some amazing tennis coaches and tennis players during my time there, including a tennis player with one leg who had more fun and a better attitude than most people with two. There were young kids who would've never been able to attend a camp like that because their family couldn't afford it but got to go because of a grant. After learning about the home lives of some of those kids, it made it quite easy to make them feel welcome and become a friend for just three short days that they would never forget.

At the end of this amazing three-day camp, the closing banquet almost *always* results in tears from both instructors and campers. I won't lie, I held back a few tears after seeing the impact this three-day camp had on some of the kids and adults who attended it. It can be hard at times, but it's extremely important to try to recognize how blessed you are and be grateful for what you have.

The directors and counselors who make this camp run are changing lives through a sport that anyone can play – and I highly encourage going there if you ever get the chance – whether you currently know how to play tennis or not.

The second event that changed my mindset occurred during my sophomore year of college as well. I came home to visit right before Thanksgiving break. My dad and I play racquetball for fun when we can and when my brother is also home. We were playing a normal game, not even a few points into it when my dad started sucking wind (more than he usually does playing with us) as he hunched over with his hands on his knees. He said it was no big deal, caught his breath, and we continued playing. One point later, he'd hardly ran around for 10 seconds and he was hunched over catching his breath again. Of course, he's one of those guys who doesn't believe anything is wrong until it actually is; which we found out a couple days later there was something *very* wrong that was causing him to lose his breath.

I went back to school after the weekend and got a call on Monday or Tuesday from my mom. He had to be taken into the hospital because his neck and chest were swelling up like nothing he had experienced before. Apparently, there was a large tumor closing in on his inferior vena cava (the large blood vessel that carries blood from the lower body into the heart) like an overweight koala bear squeezing onto a skinny tree. If he hadn't had access to a hospital in the few days that he finally decided to go in, he wouldn't have made it.

The reason his neck was swelling up was because the smaller blood vessels surrounding the heart were trying to make up for the lack of blood getting through the inferior vena cava; so they swelled, along with the tissue surrounding them. At first, they thought it was Hodgkin's lymphoma – the "less-serious" form of this cancer. Later on, he was officially diagnosed with non-Hodgkin's lymphoma (the "more-serious" form). All of this was happening, day by day, while I was off in another state.

At the time, I was basically just waiting for news each day on his condition. I was going about my business – classes, tennis practice, hanging out with friends – constantly thinking about what *could* happen.

Chemotherapy started shortly after Thanksgiving of that year, and he was wearing hats all throughout Christmas time and into spring. He and his doctors also decided to finish with radiation treatment to make sure the cancer had an even smaller chance of coming back. Five years later, he's doing very well and all of his post-treatment MRI's, blood work and checkups have been clear.

The good that came out of this whole situation was an appreciation for family and health. After my own dad's run with cancer, it seems like someone close to me each year after that has had some form of cancer as well. It's always unfortunate to hear about, but it's completely different when you or your own family member is going through it. I try not to take health for granted even more so than before, and I hope to help others not take their health for granted either. Health can change in an instant, even when that health condition has been slowly growing and affecting you internally for years or even decades before symptoms occur.

After that year, I've been able to handle situations and problems differently. The instant something bad happens or something doesn't go my way, I think, "That's alright, this could be worse." This doesn't mean I don't have the ability to be empathetic when someone else presents a situation to me that is tough for them that I think is "no big deal", I just believe everyone has the ability to control the way they react to certain situations.

Below are a few unfortunate events that have happened to me since my sophomore year of college that I had a much easier time dealing with after the two experiences explained above.

2012-2013

I finally got moved from #3 singles up to #2 singles halfway through my junior tennis season at the University of Wisconsin – Eau Claire. Finally, I thought, my hard work and improved mental game are starting to pay off. Shortly thereafter, our team was playing football for fun conditioning one afternoon. I took one wrong step at the wrong time changing directions – something I've done thousands of times – and I severely sprain my right ankle. I've sprained/rolled my ankle multiple times to a small degree, but nothing even remotely close to this. Luckily,

I was right next to the athletic training room on campus so I got helped onto a table inside right away.

I felt dizzy, nauseous, and almost as if this couldn't be real. As my ankle continued to swell, all I could think is *what perfect timing.* The year I'm starting at #1 doubles and #2 singles, my best year of tennis yet, I sprain my ankle this badly two days before a home tournament and 10 days before our team goes to play tennis in South Carolina for spring break.

I'm running through scenarios in my head of how I'm going to break the news to my parents – my dad who is still slowly on the upswing from his run with cancer, and my mom who booked the trip for both of them to come watch me play tennis on spring break for the first time. *How could this possibly get any worse one week before spring break?* The pain from my ankle made me sick, but the idea that I wasn't going to be playing the first year my parents were going to come down to watch me after my dad was recovering from cancer made me even sicker.

I got crutches from the athletic trainers and started making my way home. If you don't know what UW - Eau Claire's campus looks like, it's beautiful. A river runs through the middle of it and there is an upper and lower campus surrounded by trees and a very large staircase and hill (that most students despise, excluding me). Unfortunately, for a kid who just sprained his ankle and is on crutches, he still needs to get down the ~166-step staircase through the hilly woods to lower campus so he can get a ride home. I thought, no big deal, I'll just grab the handrails and hop down on my good leg one step at a time.

On the way down, I was so worried about hitting my bad ankle on the steps that after I reached the last step of the second staircase, I landed on the side of my "good" ankle and sprained that one too. The teammates I was with thought I was kidding as I clutched the handrail and paused for a second, saying I just landed on the outside of my other foot. I laugh at myself, mostly out of pity, wondering how this could be happening (I really did think I was coordinated still). *It's okay, hop it off, take a deep breath, that wasn't that bad, it just hurts a little bit.* So, I tried hopping on it... that was not going to happen. *Fantastic, I now have two sprained ankles 10 days before spring break.* My teammates accompanying me helped carry me down the rest of the ~140 steps and into their car before they dropped me off at home.

As funny as that might have seemed – with the odds of spraining two ankles in one day – it was one of the worst things I've personally experienced. (This was the wonderful spring that was blessed with snow as late as May 4th in Wisconsin.) So, I have two sprained ankles and am one week from leaving for spring break. I live about a mile from campus so I take a public transportation bus to and from class and I get to hobble through snow and ice on crutches with a wrapped badly sprained ankle and one "good" ankle with a brace on it. I was far from mobile.

The silver lining of this story is although I badly sprained one ankle including some nice, deep bone bruising and inflexibility that is still with me (5+ years later so far), I was still able to play doubles on spring break with my usual partner at the number one spot thanks to my coach's decision to keep us together. I couldn't move much, run, or jump, but I got to play for my parents, made the best out of the situation and still had fun nonetheless. Oh, and we ended up winning all but one of our doubles matches despite my immobility. Thanks, partner.

Summer 2013

What an amazing summer 2013 brought. I got to teach tennis, compete in a few races, and complete my summer internship at my hometown fitness center. The summer before my senior year came to an abrupt halt. I still remember this incident like it was yesterday.

I was biking home from the gym and got hit by someone who, I still believe, never looked back before opening her door into traffic. Her car door just barely hit the end of my handlebar by half an inch, sending me flying into Main Street at about 25 miles an hour. It all happened faster than I had any time to react to. I picked myself up, checked my arms and legs, looked around, and found my water bottle and bike a couple cars down.

Holy crap, that just happened and I'm okay. I looked back at the lady who opened her door, and she looked as if nothing happened, looking towards me and my bike with a perplexed look on her face. I put the chain back on my bike and hopped on thinking all was well. It was well, besides a few minor bumps and scrapes, until I pushed down on my handlebar with my left hand and felt a bit of a numb, crunching feeling.

I went to school for Kinesiology, so injuries were a part of my education and they still interest me. I moved my thumb, squeezed my fist slightly, and noticed a bit of bone where it shouldn't have been. *Okay, I either just broke my thumb – that's about 6 weeks, or it's dislocated and I need to pop it back into place.* I decided to pull on it slightly to feel what was going on inside. (I like to self-diagnose when I believe it won't hurt me further, whether advised or not.) All I felt was a little crunch, that of bone on bone, and it was clear that it was broken.

I biked home with one hand on my handlebars (I wouldn't recommend that choice either) and calmly told my mom I crashed and needed to go to the hospital because my thumb was broken (although, I was upset I had to go to the ER when homemade pizza was going in the oven).

I felt like I was another victim of extremely unfortunate luck. After all, I was about to leave for my first trip into the Boundary Waters Canoe Area Wilderness for a few days of the best fishing anyone could ask for with my best friend from high school. On top of that, my last race of the summer – the Minneapolis Duathlon of which I trained a majority of the summer for – was one week away. *Perfect #$%&ing timing again.*

After being evaluated a few times, it was decided that I was going to have surgery on it to make sure it healed properly. Hearing my surgeon say, "You *should* get full-function of your hand back" before going into surgery was one of the worst, and at the same time, most comforting, things I could've heard. *There's a chance I might not? Are you serious?* I took a deep breath and put my trust in those who were taking care of me.

Four pins and getting a cast on my way to school for my senior year was a great start to the fall. For a very brief time, I felt sorry for myself that I had to miss out on running the race, and for my friend, for missing out on our long-planned trip of fishing and camping in paradise. Once I was able to get back to the reality of the situation, I got through it by looking on the bright side.

The *very* silver lining: I was thrown from my bike into a very busy street, which rarely has a block-long break with no cars in either lane, without a helmet (I wear one now), and I didn't hit my head on anything. My bike got a few scratches, but still works fine. I didn't get run over by a car after tumbling several feet having no idea what was going on. My phone and tennis racket in the outside pocket of the backpack I was wearing both remained unbroken. I broke the thumb on my non-dominant hand, so I was able to write normally during school. All I was left with was a disappointing end to my summer, a missed race, a missed camping trip, a missed senior fall season of tennis and a broken thumb. I was, and still am, extremely fortunate and thankful that I didn't end up with further injuries.

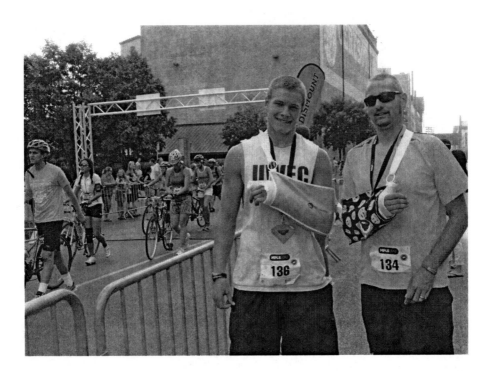

Winter 2014

This is a short story, I promise. Two weeks into my first season coaching the girls' varsity hockey team, another coach and I were playing around with the players on the ice. One player tried to lift my stick for the puck, missed, and hit me right above the eye. It didn't really hurt so I laughed and looked up at the girl who hit me and asked if I was bleeding. The girl I asked had a reaction that was reason enough to go check it out in the mirror.

A swollen, bloody, and colorful mark above my left eye, sweet! I went to the hospital, didn't end up needing stitches, and came back for the rest of practice with a funny-looking bandage above my eye. After practice, we had our first parent meeting in which I jokingly informed the parents not to mess with their daughters unless they want to end up looking like me.

Some coaches might have been upset or angry at the player for being so careless with their stick around a coach during such a light-hearted game of keep-away, but all I could think was *thank you for not hitting me in the eye.* One centimeter lower and I might not be seeing with both eyes. Once again, I'm unlucky enough to get another injury, but on the bright side, I'm lucky enough to still see out of both eyes. Also, I no longer play keep-away from the players before practice.

Health Tip to Try

When an unfortunate event or circumstance happens to you or is present in your life, immediately search for the "silver lining" or bright side of the situation, and make the best of it. If you can focus on the positive –like being able to still play tennis, having your dominant hand, not cracking your head on the street, or still being able to see out of both eyes – rather than the negative – I'm injured at a really bad time, I'm missing half my senior tennis season, I can't use my left hand, I have a small scar above my eyebrow – you'll be able to stay positive throughout that tough time a lot easier than if you just focus on the negative aspects of the situation.

Stay positive, and positivity will fill your day. Stay negative, and negativity will fill your day. Often times, there can be a positive to a negative situation. Your ability to see the good during the bad can enlighten your mindset and your life.

We all have that one friend, coworker or family member who always seems to be complaining about something going on in their life. You may see them once a day, week or month; but when you do, you know there's only one tone to the conversation – and it's a negative one.

Unfortunately for these people, they don't usually realize they're doing it. It's only clear to them when someone else points it out each and every time they hear the negativity. I have a friend who struggles with this problem. She has a very short fuse and a weak tolerance to things not going according to plan. When I point out what she's getting frustrated or mad about she usually responds, "Yeah... I know, I know. It's not that big of a deal." But it *is* that big of a deal.

I believe everyone has the capacity to change their mindset if they commit to it. It can't be a half-assed effort like you're going to try a "juice cleanse" for a week to drop 10 lbs, only to gain back 15 lbs two weeks later. It has to be slow and steady. It has to be consistent – reminding yourself every single day and multiple times per day what you have to be happy about when things don't seem to be going your way.

The people who don't have reasons to be happy at any certain point during the day are spending too much time focusing on reasons to be unhappy. Here's a scenario (pay attention to my parentheses):

Betty is talking to her friend (whom she is able to exercise with 5 days per week) at the gym (that gives her an insurance kickback so her membership is $15/month) while they casually float around on the elliptical on level 2 out of 25. She's explaining how she's had the *worst* day ever. First, she got stuck in traffic (in her BMW) on her way to work (where she has a full-time job, with benefits, and makes $60,000/year) where she ended up arriving 10 minutes late (nobody noticed her slight tardiness). In her eyes, this day was already off to a bad start. She forgot her lunch (which she has no problem affording) on the dining room table because who hasn't done that at least once or twice (she can order food to be delivered to her office) and is pissed about the extra 10 minutes she took to prepare it, now only to go to waste. Around 2:30pm, she spills coffee creamer (which her office provides for employees daily) on her black work pants (that her employer paid for) and is forced to change into her black yoga pants she's planning on working out in ($100 Lulu's, of course) for the rest of the work day.

Betty sees this day as a disaster. But if you read my notes, you can see she has a *lot* to be thankful for in the first place. Obviously, this day didn't go as smoothly as it could've, but with a positive mindset and good attitude she too could see the bright side and be happy with what she has, even when things don't go according to plan.

Motivation

*"It has been my observation that most people get ahead
during the time that others waste."*

-Henry Ford

Where to Begin

Evaluating yourself is key to learning how to stay motivated. Below is an evaluation of your own motivation that covers a few basic areas.

1.   What gets/keeps you motivated to do well in your career?

What is one barrier?

What is one solution to overcome that barrier?

2.   What gets/keeps you motivated to eat healthy?

What is one barrier?

What is one solution to overcome that barrier?

3.   What gets/keeps you motivated to exercise?

What is one barrier?

What is one solution to overcome that barrier?

4. What gets/keeps you motivated to build new relationships and keep the ones you already have?

What is one barrier?

What is one solution to overcome that barrier?

There are many more questions you could ask yourself when it comes to evaluating what motivates you. The areas of your life that need constant sources of motivation the most are the first aspects you may need to focus on.

Aspects of your life that are easy to maintain motivation for or come second nature to you (like exercising and eating healthy *now* for me) don't need to be focused on as much. Do you lose motivation to exercise after one week? Do you lose motivation to keep friends close because you lack the time to stay in touch? Do you have trouble finding motivation to move up in your current career field?

As a Precision Nutrition (PN) coach, I frequently will ask the "5 Why's" to my clients. It's an easy way to get to the bottom of someone's motivation. It'll teach me and the client what their greatest motivator is – the "deep" reason behind their actions.

Ask yourself the "5 Why's", think about each answer for a minute as if you *were* doing PN coaching, and see what you come up with. (Precision Nutrition coaching is a habit-based way of coaching that focuses on slowly changing lifestyle and eating habits to make weight loss, athletic performance, and day-to-day eating and living easier. PN is the founder of the "5 Why's".) For example:

Why do you want to do Precision Nutrition coaching?

Client: Because I'm sick and tired of being sick and tired.

Why is that reason for taking action important to you?

Client: Because I've been slogging through life long enough, I know I'm not getting any younger and I want to *feel* better.

And why is *that* reason important?

Client: Because my energy levels and motivation keep me from achieving my goals and being as happy as I know I can be each day.

And what difference will changing make?

Client: I will be able to be more productive in all aspects of my life – family, work, health, etc. and be less stressed out about what I'm not accomplishing because of my lack of energy.

And why will that previous thing matter to you?

Client: Because I want to feel fulfilled at the end of the day. I want to grow as a person and have a positive impact on those around me.

Wow. Who thought asking repetitive questions could reveal an underlying motive like that? If you don't get this activity to reveal anything major for you and you *did* think deeply about each "why", not a problem. You can also try changing the first "why" question to reflect something you want to change. For example:

Why do you want to exercise more?

Client: Because I'm starting to realize I can't keep up with my kids, and I want to be able to be active with them.

Why is that reason for taking action important to you?

Client: Because I want to be present in their lives, and if they're active, I should be active too.

And why is *that* reason important?

Client: Because I see plenty of other parents being active with their kids up until they graduate high school, and I want to be that parent.

And what difference will changing make?

Client: I will be in better shape for my own good, but also to set a good example for my kids so hopefully they develop the habit of being active as they get older and leave home too.

And why will that previous thing matter to you?

Client: Because I want my kids to look up to me, learn positive things from me, and to live a healthy life after they're gone. I also need to stay healthy to be *able* to watch them grow and live a healthy life.

Self-reflection is a useful tool and can get you to think about your motives in a way you haven't done before. Writing things down also makes them a lot more concrete. Besides getting behind your own motives and understanding them better, setting small, realistic goals to reach your desired outcome will help you stay motivated and feel successful along the way.

Try to set a goal for yourself each month. That goal can be anything: I want to cook healthier meals, I want to walk my dog more, I want to get noticed for my hard work in my career. Goals are easy to set. The problem arises when goals are not tracked and evaluated. You can set all the goals you want, but without a plan and consistent progress checks, that goal is going to be difficult to achieve.

Just like in Strategy One, you can create a SMART goal for just about anything. Follow the model, or a similar one, in Strategy One and keep it in a safe place. Hanging your SMART goal on your bulletin board in your office or at home where it is easy to see will help reinforce what you're working towards and you can consistently track and re-evaluate how your progress is coming along. If SMART goals help keep you motivated, then by all means use them as much as possible.

How I Stay Motivated

Even someone who believes he's got his motivation under control (like me) can slip up once in a while. Intrinsic motivation and extrinsic motivation are two different types of motivation that can help motivate someone in different aspects of his or her life. I personally use both from time to time and I know they both have pros and cons.

Individuals with intrinsic motivation can motivate themselves just by their thoughts and feelings about bettering themselves in some way. They don't need outside help. They don't need a group of people to exercise with. They might decide they're going to run a faster mile next month just for the sake of improving their mile time and getting faster and plan to run four times per week to accomplish that goal.

People who need extrinsic motivation require an outside source or influence to provide their motivation. They might lift weights just because they enjoy getting compliments about their physique. They may only attend exercise classes because there are guaranteed to be other people around them exercising too. They might put a dollar in a jar every time they complete a workout and buy themselves a new pair of running shoes once they reach a certain amount to continue the extrinsic motivation pathway (which is a great strategy, by the way).

Combining intrinsic and extrinsic motivation might be seen in the individual who likes the way they feel after exercising in the morning (intrinsic – it is motivating to exercise because it makes their physical and mental self feel better) and they also exercise because they need to stay in shape to teach exercise classes at their gym (extrinsic because an outside source – the people who attend the exercise class – motivate them to stay in top shape and present a positive example).

Whichever type of motivation works better for you is the type you want to capitalize on. If you function better with one type of motivation, I would also encourage you to seek motivation from the opposite type to test the waters. This can open your eyes to more sources of motivation that may or may not work for you. Even if you already feel like you're well off being intrinsically motivated, finding someone who pushes you in the gym (who becomes a source of extrinsic motivation for you to increase strength just like they are) can add to your own sources of motivation and increase your success as well.

Losing Motivation, and Getting it Back

Losing motivation happens to everyone. For some, it might happen for a day or two, for others, it might be six months to a year. I've lost motivation for short periods of time many times before but have always managed to get back on track. There are a few things that you can do to help you forget your slip up and move on.

1. **Accept the fact that you have slipped up**. You may have missed two straight weeks of exercising, eaten fast food four times in one week, or have gotten into an unproductive slump at work. Remember, you're a human and humans aren't perfect, so don't expect to be.

2. This is the most important part: **forgive and forget**. You need to move on without dwelling on how long you slipped up, how major the slip up was, how much weight you gained, or what it *might* mean for the future. You can change your present and future and you can start doing that as soon as you forget about the past.

3. **Find your motivation again**. Either revert back to the source of motivation that works best for you, or, if this is the seventh time you've slipped up for the same reasons, then try a different source of motivation to help keep you on track (or ask yourself the "5 Why's" again). If something isn't working, you have to try something new.

Like I mentioned earlier, our health is often a game of guess-and-check. If something doesn't work for you, try something else!

There are other reasons one might start to lose motivation. An athlete might lose motivation because they get "burnt out" of the sport. They might practice too much and get too little rest. They might be sick of their coaches/teammates/parents getting on them for screwing up or for putting pressure on them to perform.

A stay-at-home mom might lose motivation for multiple different things because it's so much easier to make excuses when you have a child to raise and take care of. They can keep putting off their "start" to a healthy lifestyle again until the child is older; soon enough the child is two years old, the mother hasn't changed a bit, and she wonders what happened. If being healthy for your children (so you can play with them, keep up with them, watch them grow older, etc.) isn't motivating enough for parents to take care of themselves, I don't know what is.

When it comes to the term "overreaching", it is usually referring to exercise but I'm including it with motivation because it can be a big motivation-killer. Overreaching describes increasing the intensity/

frequency/volume of your training or exercise in order to improve. You could even apply overreaching to other aspects outside of exercise such as trying to change too many eating habits at once in order to make quicker progress.

Some people don't believe something somewhat similar – overtraining – is a real thing. Overtraining refers to the feelings of sluggishness, regression, and loss of energy/motivation from training to the point where you don't want to train anymore and you may even develop overuse injuries from the activity you're performing. For a small select number of people, they might push themselves to the edge constantly and never experience overtraining. For a majority of people who start an exercise or fitness program, this becomes all too real.

Imagine you haven't exercised in nine months. You lose your breath walking up the stairs from your basement (because that's where you keep your frozen pizzas) to your living room and you can hardly carry in two bags of groceries from the car because your arms can't hold the weight.

You decide it's time to get in shape because your cousin's wedding is in 8 weeks. So, you start lifting weights three days per week and running two miles (because who can't handle a little two-mile jog?) on your non-lifting days. The first four days are fantastic; you feel slightly sore from your new lifting program and energized from running and think this is going great. You continue the same schedule of lifting and running every other day for another week.

Soon, you start to feel consistently sore every day of the week in the same areas on your body and your two-mile running time slows by 1 minute and 30 seconds. Your appetite wanes and your sleep quality starts to diminish. You think, *I can't keep this up anymore; I need to stop* (so you do).

As quickly as this great start to a healthy lifestyle came, it is now gone. You haven't exercised in a week and aren't sure what to do in fear that the same feelings will come back again – and you *really* don't want to feel overly sore or tired. This is a perfect example of overreaching/overtraining to the point of losing motivation to continue. This is not the goal.

Health Tip to Try

Keep track of how you feel (maybe a 1-10 scale, 10 being fantastic), once a day, once you begin or alter your diet/fitness habits. This could be cutting out or adding in a different type of food or increasing the number of days you run or lift weights each week. If you notice a decline in your mood, appetite, sleep quality or performance, dial down the adjustment you made and record how you feel again. Aim for an 8 or higher each day. Guess and check!

The goal is to improve at a steady enough pace that this cycle doesn't occur. Ever heard of yo-yo dieting? You most likely have and are now aware that "yo-yo training/exercising" is a real thing too and it's just as challenging as yo-yo dieting. The goal is for your exercise program to never make you feel like you're run down, your sleep suffers, you're irritable and tired, and you actually don't want to start exercising again. This reason, among others, is why so many people fail at keeping themselves motivated.

Of course, people are going to be sore post-training for a few weeks when starting an exercise program after taking a long time off – that's inevitable and normal. The soreness will decrease as the consistency increases. It should be the top priority to be able to keep your motivation high when starting any part of your healthy lifestyle from ground zero because if you lose motivation, you will often lose hope.

Start with something *so easy* that you know you're going to succeed at it. Remember the SMART goal scale of 1-10. If you set out to do something and you ask yourself on a scale of 1 (I can't do that) to 10 (there's no way I'll fail), you should be at a 9 or a 10 on that scale. If you aren't, make the task easier until you are.

Jarod loves exercising hard but he runs into problems when he exercises too hard. Sometimes, he takes a few weeks off from exercise because of a busy schedule before a week-long vacation and he comes back and jumps in like he never left. After returning from vacation, he plans on hitting the gym hard for the next two weeks straight, vowing to "get back on track".

Jarod is great at motivating himself to exercise but loses motivation when he doesn't see the quick results he wants. He reads magazines and watches videos online that explain how simple it is to lose body fat by doing certain workouts and certain lifts. When he goes hard in the gym, he expects his triceps to be cut, his biceps to bulge, and his calves to rip jeans before the month is up.

After a couple weeks of a healthier diet and hard work and no immediate results to show for it (besides you know, feeling better, having more energy, better sleep, etc.), he loses motivation to continue his hard workout schedule and once again stops exercising and eating well for a few weeks.

Motivating yourself can be a difficult task. What Jarod learned after realizing what his problem was is that it's better to find a happy medium that you can maintain (while forgetting about the quick results everyone wants) that doesn't cause you to be a yo-yo dieter or exerciser – even if it's far less intense than you think it "should" be. Once he adjusted his workout schedule to a more long-term friendly amount of four to five days per week with two to three full rest days – and his diet – so he was allowed a few treats every week, he started to see and feel the results he wanted after about 6-8 weeks.

You need to realize the body is an intricate organism that will rarely react exactly how you expect it to, especially if you're comparing your *progress* to someone else's *results*. Find the right exercise plan and amount of motivation that will keep you wanting to come back for more week after week, month after month, and year after year. Eventually, you'll see the results you're looking for.

Lifestyle Habits

"Quality means doing it right when no one is looking."
-Henry Ford

Where to Begin

Lifestyle habits are what separate the generally healthy from the persistently ill. Habits keep the body and mind on the right track. Habits stay consistent when life can be constantly inconsistent. People who practice positive lifestyle habits are the ones who find staying "healthy" effortless. People who don't practice positive lifestyle habits are the ones who are frequently sick, tired, injured, or fighting a medical condition such as diabetes, high blood pressure, or high cholesterol. They might have no idea what they're doing wrong that's causing those problems or what they could easily change to help fight them. To me, a healthier lifestyle is one that keeps you on the right side of the health continuum and is *easy* to maintain; so it stays on the right side without undue effort.

Sleep

Sufficient sleep is well known to be good and the reasons for this are clear. Sleep allows your mind and body to recover and repair itself. Sleep has been shown to solidify memories from the previous day and better allow the use of those memories later on (1). Sleep loss can lead to impaired cognitive and behavioral performance. Furthermore, during long periods without sleep and circadian phase misalignment due to inconsistent sleep patterns, cognitive performance has also been shown to decrease. In one study performed in 2012, sleep loss exhibited its primary effect on feelings of sleepiness during the day (duh) and a decrease in the ability to sustain attention to tasks (2). Lack of sleep equals lack of focus and we all know what it feels like to have trouble concentrating and keeping our attention focused on the task in front of us whether that be operating some type of machinery, presenting to a group, taking a test, or just reading. When it comes to health and fitness, this point is relevant if you think about the amount of mental focus it takes to go to the grocery store or out to eat and be able to make the right choices for your goals, or going to the gym and having a solid, focused workout. Mental fog from lack of sleep can lead to an array of poor, impulsive decisions.

There are exceptions to the results of such studies of course, and I think we all know that one friend or colleague who can run on 2-3 hours less of sleep each night when most of us feel tired, slow and groggy on that same amount of sleep. The amount of sleep required to feel "rested" can vary from person to person just like any other interpersonal characteristic.

One simple way to find out how much sleep for you is optimal is to try to get into a schedule of going to bed and waking up at the same time every day. By waking up at the same time each day (yes, perhaps even on weekends), you can experiment with the amount of sleep you get by adjusting your bedtime. If you're going to attempt this, I would suggest trying a certain bedtime for more than one night at a time to give your body a chance to get used to it. Going to bed at a different time each night makes it near impossible to get a consistent number of hours of sleep per night and especially to notice how you feel after a certain amount of sleep. For example, I feel great if I get between 7.5 and 8.5 hours of sleep per night. Getting much less or much more than that I feel less rested and less energized than I do within that certain window. Once again, guess and check.

For those of you who can't make it to sleep at the same time each night for certain reasons (family, kids, health, etc.), one of the first places you need to look to help this problem is your time-management skills. Spending 30 extra minutes surfing the web or 90 extra minutes watching TV can sneak up quickly and can easily screw up the regular schedule of going to sleep around the same time each night. If you've tried everything you can think of on your own and your sleep still suffers, consider seeing a specialist to see if there's another reason why you can't get quality sleep.

Creating a daily schedule might be the trick to get on track. The most important time to manage your schedule is likely the evening because that is when most of the activities after work or school are occurring (if you have a family or regular day-time job). Steps you can take to improve your time-management in the evenings include, but are not limited to:

1. **Have a plan for dinner** – what you're eating, if you have the ingredients, if someone needs to go to the store, how long it takes to prepare and eat, who's preparing it – all need to be accounted for to allow time for dinner. Sometimes, the best dinners are ones that can be kept warm and eaten by members of the family when it's convenient for them on busy nights. Refer back to Strategy Two if you need to.

2. **Is your favorite show** that you *must* watch on tonight? Can you record it and save up to 15 minutes of your time by fast-forwarding commercials? Can you eat dinner while it's showing to save time that particular night? Clean while it's on? Too busy to work out during the day, but can you perform exercises during the show or on the commercials? Too much TV is one of the biggest culprits for loss of sleep and productivity.

3. **Know who has what activity/meeting/event**, how long the event is, and how they're getting to and from there (if you have children). Planning rides and car-pooling can save a lot of time and hassle. If you live in an area where it's safe for your child to use a bike for transportation, give them some freedom (along with yourself) and invest in a bike for them.

4. As mentioned earlier, **know what time you want to be in bed** by so you can help yourself plan up until that time. Try preparing for bed ~20-30 minutes before that set time. That way, when those little meaningless nighttime tasks present themselves and catch your attention, you've got a little time to spare.

Sitting vs. Standing

I fully believe you need to spend less time sitting. Believe it or not, I probably wrote 90% of this book standing rather than sitting. Although you might be thinking, *wow, this is awful, I don't think I want to stand while I do anything now,* I urge you to try standing more often and while doing things you would normally do sitting like reading, studying, work related tasks or even eating. Standing desks can range anywhere from home-made (my favorite) to $100-$500+. They come adjustable, have multiple platforms, and there are even desks with a treadmill right underneath them if you want to get crazy.

A review conducted in 2011 found that total sedentary time was negatively associated with cardiovascular risk factors and that breaking up prolonged sitting/sedentary time was positively associated with those same risk factors (3). More intervention studies are needed before we fully understand the reasoning behind those findings, but if breaking up prolonged periods of sitting by just standing more often or moving around every 20-30 minutes on a regular basis can have those positive outcomes among others then why not give it a try?

Getting up and walking around and/or stretching every 20-30 minutes if you work at a desk can make a big difference in your health, posture, focus, and productivity. If you work a desk job, there are three things I would recommend trying for one week straight to see how your body, energy, and focus feel:

1. Stand up and walk around the office (maybe 1 minute of walking) every 30-45 minutes.
2. Stretch the front of your hip and your core by performing the following stretch once every 1-2 hours (or every other walking break to make it simple) for 20-30 seconds per side.
   a. Assume a lunge stance with your front left knee bent about 90 degrees, and back right leg straight. Reach up with your right hand as high as you can, push your hips down towards the ground, and lean to your left while letting out a long, deep breath. To heighten the stretch of the hip flexor of your back leg, contract the glute of your back leg as well. Repeat on the other side.
3. Stretch your chest/anterior shoulder.
   a. Stand in a doorway and place both of your elbows or hands against the doorframe. Slightly lean forward through the doorway until you feel a stretch in the front of your shoulders and your chest. Hold for 20-30 seconds and repeat 1-3 times.

Tight, rolled forward shoulders and tight quads and hips occurring from too much sitting can lead to many different physical ailments and inconsistencies. Standing while working or taking frequent walk breaks can help keep your core and posture strong and help to avoid back pain while simultaneously burning more calories over the course of a day than while sitting for long periods of time (4).

One study conducted by Bailey et al. in 2015 found that even when breaking up prolonged periods of sitting time by getting up every 20 minutes and briefly walking, one can increase their total daily energy expenditure along with decreasing their post-meal blood sugar spike without increasing their overall appetite. Even more interestingly, they found that relative energy intake (calorie consumption) was even *higher* in the test group that spent the entire 5-hour period sitting when they consumed a meal at the end compared to the people who briefly walked every 20 minutes. At the end of the day, the sedentary people ended up moving less and eating more; that's a double whammy (5).

In addition to the benefits of standing/moving frequently instead of prolonged sitting as a great lifestyle habit, walking extra every chance you get (if you aren't in a huge hurry) can be another habit that adds up your daily caloric burn. Park further back in the parking lot, take the long way around the building to get to your office, walk an extra five minutes after lunch with a friend or coworker, or take the stairs. It all adds up to more daily energy expenditure and non-exercise activity thermogenesis (NEAT) and keeps your body in an "active" mode. If you want some extra entertainment or simply missed the news heading "sitting is the new smoking", Google the phrase and read up. If you're really interested in knowing just about everything there is to know about the detriments of sitting to the body, check out Kelly Starrett's *Deskbound*.

Health Tip to Try

Stand while performing a task (like reading, studying, working, or eating) at least 3 consecutive days/times and see how you feel physically and mentally. Try standing on a foot-massaging ball or roll a tennis ball under the bottom of your feet as you stand as well.

If you're already active but would be considered an "exercising couch potato", which is 100% a lifestyle habit or a combination of several habits, consider this:

When you exercise consistently, your body will eventually begin to adapt by increasing your cardiovascular efficiency, strength, and endurance; increasing your muscular strength; increasing bone/joint health; and decreasing your fat mass to name a few. When you're an exercising couch potato, your sedentary lifestyle decreases your lean body mass and increases fat mass; it decreases your bone density; it decreases your flexibility; and it decreases your muscular strength, endurance, and power, to name a few. All of these factors are also either bettered or worsened depending on the diet you consume.

When you're consistently sitting or being sedentary the majority of your day, whether you're exercising regularly or not, you are, in a way, holding yourself back. I would equate the exercising couch potato to an overweight and inactive individual trying to make their way up the wrong side of an escalator. They're getting some work done during that short burst of effort to climb a few steps, but if they take even a few moments (in the real world, several days) off, the hard work they put in to gain several vertical feet completely disappears and they're back to square one the minute they let up. The only thing they gained is the experience of starting and quitting, which hopefully this time they learned from.

The unfortunate thing about poor lifestyle habits is that they can work to undue your exercise efforts. A consistent exercise regimen can give you slow and steady noticeable gains over the course of 4-12 weeks. Unfortunately, if you take just a few weeks completely off, your progress can deflate back to square one (or, in the short-term, back to where you started as a trained individual just 4-12 weeks ago). That is one of the reasons why lifestyle habits are so important and staying consistent is going to make or break your long-term progress. Anyone who's taken a solid 2-3 weeks off running or lifting when they regularly have been doing both knows how fast your physical conditioning can regress.

Drinking Water

Something I greatly dislike about the common water recommendation of "8 glasses per day" is its oversimplification. How big are your "glasses" or cups compared to mine? How much do you weigh? How active are you on the job/during the day? How much do you exercise/sweat? What kind of food are you eating during the day? What medications are you taking? Do you drink coffee? All of these questions and many more can change that amount of "8 glasses per day" for any given person.

For anyone who is an athlete, exercises each day, or competes in events such as races or sporting events, this recommendation can be quite misleading. I know a *ton* of athletes and consistently active people who think this recommendation is good for them (even if they don't already reach it) when in reality, the amount that they might sweat on any given day needs to be replaced and this recommendation just isn't going to cut it.

I am not going to give you the formula for how much fluid you need to drink based on the water weight you lost during exercise (although you can find it after a little searching if interested) because for the general population and also the physically active population, it's not necessary to obsess over. A great goal to have when consuming water each day, like I stated in Strategy Two, is to consume half your body weight, in ounces of water, per day. This, like any other recommendation I might give you or you might hear, is dependent upon the person. Maybe for your specific activity level this is too much or not enough, but it's likely going to get you closer to proper hydration than the generic "8 glasses per day". This leads me to my next "Health Tip to Try", which is more of a "live by this each and every day" suggestion that makes hydrating correctly simple.

Health Tip to Try

Look at the color of your urine each time you go. Many people know that dark colored and strong-smelling urine is a sign of dehydration, but most of them don't look to see what their urine looks like each time they go. This is by far the easiest and most hassle-free way to see if you're hydrated. Aim (pun not intended) for a very light yellow colored urine. If your urine is on the darker side, you know you need to drink more water. Simple as that.

The other ugly side of dehydration is its effects on bowel movements. Dehydration has been shown to increase the likelihood of constipation and disruption of normal bowel movements (6). If you have trouble with bowel movements or they're as inconsistently timed, passed, or solid as your water consumption habits, your dehydration may be the issue.

Dehydration isn't the only point of concern when looking at your bowel movements (if you want to know more about what your bowel movements can say about your health, ask your doctor or do a little digging on your own). Your diet is arguably the number one factor leading to the ease and consistency of your bowel movements. By consistency, I don't just mean going at nearly the same time each day. I mean the color, the shape, the solidity, and the size. These factors, among others, can be signs of problems going on inside your digestive tract that could be due to your diet or fluid intake, or due to something more complicated.

To make it simple, having bowel movements that are of consistent shape (long and oval shaped), size (depends on the person), solidity (semi-soft), and color (light to dark brown) are sought. If you believe you exercise consistently (another factor affecting bowel movements), eat a healthy diet containing enough fiber, and consume enough fluids but don't have "normal" bowel movements as described, you may want to consider seeing a doctor.

Drinking enough water is simple if you can follow these three steps:

1. **Have a nice (preferably BPA free) water bottle** that you're not ashamed to be seen with in public and carry it with you everywhere you go. No, carrying it with you empty does not count.
2. **Drink water at regular intervals.** This is important to avoid going 2-3 hours without drinking any and then trying to chug 15oz of dreaded room temperature water pre-workout to make up for it. Drinking at regular intervals, sometimes even when you're not thirsty if you know you're going to be exercising soon, will prevent that catch-up from needing to happen.
   a. To get used to this idea, consider making a few marks on your water bottle (or a cleaned milk jug, etc.) with corresponding times of day. Watch the clock and see if you can stay on track with your daily goal.
3. **Drink an entire glass of cool water upon waking up.** That means before coffee, eggs, oats, etc. This is an awesome habit to start your day with to get on the right track to normal hydration.

If plain water is unappealing to you, try adding lemon or lime, berries, cinnamon, or mint to your bottle. There are now plenty of bottles out there that have a nice little container on the inside that allows you to make your own naturally flavored water without making a mess or getting a mint leaf stuck in your teeth right before an important job interview.

My opinion on powdered flavored beverage sweeteners such as Crystal Light, Gatorade, and the like is basically just to minimize your intake and use them on an as-needed basis. If they get you to drink your water then great, that's better than being dehydrated each day and it's a step in the right direction, but eventually you're going to want to wean off of them (and use them sparingly) to save money in the long run and increase your intake of plain water (with no additives, artificial sweeteners, or artificial colors) if nothing else.

If you don't really like water by itself and find it very difficult to drink enough each day, try a few different sweeteners that are either sugar free or very low in sugar (<2g per 8 fluid ounces) but only use half of the recommended amount to mix in. If flavor is what you're after, this will still give you plenty of flavor along with minimizing the amount of extra artificial sweeteners or sugar you're consuming each day, not to mention it will save you money in the long run again.

If you are trying to lose fat and maintain lean muscle mass for a specific reason, are following an intense exercise regime or are on a low-calorie diet, consider trying branched chain amino acids (BCAA's) as a flavor-enhancer in your water. They'll add flavor as well as some extra amino acids (which you also likely consume in your diet in smaller amounts, so they aren't completely necessary) that will aid recovery from exercise and work to maintain your lean body mass.

Aging

If you paid attention during the exercise strategy, you know how important exercise and resistance training are as you age. Lifestyle habits that are either good or bad will almost invariably affect you later in life.

The bad part about lifestyle habits is they're hard to break and most people don't pay much attention to them unless their body finally folds under the pressure (like with type II diabetes). Besides maintaining/building lean body mass and keeping body fat in check as you age, I believe the second most important reason for consistent exercise is for bone and joint health. If you become overweight, there are many different avenues you can take to try to get your weight back down to a healthy range. If you develop osteoporosis at the age of 45, you're in for a long and basically unwinnable battle for the rest of your life. You will become fracture-prone, and your risk of serious injury like breaking your hip during a fall (or any other bone) will increase.

There are circumstances that may be out of your control or different now than they were when you were younger (like girls/women not really playing sports or lifting weights back in the 1950's or '60's like they do today), in which case you may have been out of luck at that time because research on the effects of exercise on bone mineral density wasn't there like it is today.

Below is a story about my grandmother who grew up during that timeframe when women and exercise/sports didn't go together and what her lifestyle habits (whether in or out of her control) have set her up for as she ages.

The first story I can remember about my grandma that really got me thinking happened when I was about 10 years old. My mom happened to mention how thankful she was for her current health and informed me that she had to go help her mom because she was bending over to grab something out of her freezer (think a bag of frozen peas) and she fractured one of her ribs upon lifting it and needed immediate attention. I was too young to have any idea why something like that might happen besides bad luck, but now stories like these just add to my interest in wanting to help people (women, especially) learn about the benefits of exercise.

The second story happened when she had her knee replaced right around 2012. Picture yourself as a surgeon.

I walk into the operating room that is staffed and awaiting my arrival to begin a knee replacement. The incision is made and I can see the muscle and bony structures of the knee that I'm about to replace. After some work is done, I grab the largest piece of her new knee, the femoral component, and my assistant hands me the "hammer" that I will use to insert it into her femur. After one tap, I drop the hammer, steady myself, and use my hands to push the component straight into her femur. I've never felt bone so porous as to be able to drive the rod into the bone with just the use of my hands.

The surgeon said if her bones were any softer, they'd probably turn to dust. Once you have osteoporosis this bad (or even half as bad) there really isn't anything you can do, that we now know of, to reverse the damage done. Lifestyle intervention can help you hold onto or decrease the reduction of bone density over time if you start early and maintain, but unless you hope to undergo the procedure Wolverine had, you're out of luck.

The last two stories have to do with exercise and joint health. My grandma gets out and about when she can and she's still able to maintain her home with a little help from friends and family. In the past, I've also shown her a few exercises she can do with a resistance band for her core, legs and arms at home that she has been doing her best to complete 2-3 days per week.

She decided to go to a stretching class that was specifically for older adults. She had not been to a stretching class before and most of the stretches were done either sitting on the ground or with the assistance of a chair. Unfortunately, her body wasn't accustomed to holding the positions she was moving into and after one class, she ended up with a fractured hip. Yes, a fractured hip from attending a *stretching* class geared towards older adults.

Near the same time, she also had recently started going to the gym (because the membership is free which I think is fantastic to get this population more active) to use the NuStep and to try walking on a treadmill. The NuStep was good for her and she enjoyed it, but sitting too long hurt her back, so she decided to give the treadmill a try. As you know, if you turn the treadmill on so the track can speed up (or slow down when you're done) to your preferred walking speed while you're standing on the side of the treadmill, you have to have your feet about 2.5ft apart before you step on. Just from this wide stance alone, her hips came out of alignment before she could step on, she was immediately in a good deal of pain, her patience was up, and that was the end of her 45-second treadmill-walking career. Talk about having a short list of exercise options.

These stories aren't meant to scare you. They're meant to give you an idea of what life can look like later on if you don't take your health seriously while you still have *some* control over it. That also means just paying attention to the way you look shouldn't be your only priority when it comes to choosing exercise. Your muscle, bone, and cardiovascular strength should all be considered as well.

Have a Hobby (or Two or Three)

I believe having hobbies is good for several reasons and that there are too many things to do and to explore on this great earth for anyone to ever be bored. Your hobbies might depend on factors such as how much time you have, what your interests are, where you live and how much money you choose to spend on your personal activities.

Some of my favorite hobbies include playing the piano, bicycling, lifting weights, reading, playing sports and drawing. Notice how none of these hobbies are mind-numbing and sedentary activities like watching TV shows online for hours on end. I like them because they are active or they challenge my mind or skills in a different way.

Hobbies can challenge your brain in ways that your normal day-to-day life can't. For example, playing a musical instrument or writing your own music is going to challenge the brain in a vastly different way than playing the same video game over and over again (although video games can be great for hand-eye coordination and imagination). Hobbies can keep you active and away from the couch if yours include outdoor activities or activities you can do with friends such as tennis, volleyball, hiking, or mountain biking. Hobbies can allow you to branch out, meet new people, and experience new things. Hobbies can be a conversation starter with a stranger. Hobbies can also be a channel for de-stressing yourself.

Whatever your hobby involves doing, work to become better at it. This is an opportunity for personal growth and development that isn't going to happen on its own. Whatever your hobby is, you can become better through practice, add to your life's excitement and productivity and learn more about that hobby and see other peoples' perspectives on it to help you grow. To grow is to improve, and improvement is usually the goal, isn't it?

Brighten Other People's Day

Being kind is very underrated. Please and thank you, sure, they're nice, but do you remember the people in your life who ask you about your day, how your weekend was, or how your family is doing? I certainly don't remember the people who don't as much as the ones who do. A smile at a friend or coworker, a wave to a stranger driving by, or holding the door open for someone you don't know can have an impact on their day that you have no idea occurred.

It is like walking into a bank and being genuinely moved by how polite, smiley, and interested the tellers are about your (a complete stranger) day. I've never been greeted, talked to, or said goodbye to as enthusiastically as I am when just walking inside my bank. If your bank isn't as spectacular as mine, you're really missing out on a great five-minute errand. These people are the epitome of kindness in everyday life that has the ability to rub off on those who experience it.

If people acted like that, not to be successful at their job position, but in everyday life, imagine how everyone's mood could change. No cranky customers telling you what you're doing wrong and never what you're doing right. No ungrateful co-workers who don't notice how much you help them each and every day. It's probably a little far-fetched, but one can dream.

Health Tip to Try

When you encounter someone (not a close friend or family member) in your daily life, ask them how their day is going rather than just nodding or saying "hi" and walking by. You might be amazed at how good you can feel inside and out by taking some interest in those around you.

Balance

Balance was going to be an entire strategy when I was outlining this project, but frankly, I don't think I could come up with enough information regarding balance nor do I want to make you read something that might just be rambling when the entire goal of this book is to inform you about balance.

When considering the information in each strategy, there is no cut-and-dry way to go about applying it to your life so it works without any setbacks regarding your diet, exercise, stress, outlook, motivation, or lifestyle habits. Everyone will have some type of setback for whatever reason; injury, traveling, family matters, health, loss of motivation, marriage, kids and the list goes on.

Balance comes in handy when you know you're going to have a setback or are in the middle of one (which *will* happen). I know I'm going to continue to have them throughout my life and I'm OK with that. That's one of the reasons why I find myself to be quite successful. I don't lose focus or get flustered when things don't go according to plan because while I'm making a plan, I'm already *planning* on encountering a setback or two. There's no surprise for regressing or failing, it's all just part of the realistic process. Accept the fact that success isn't a straight line or one-way street and you're halfway there.

Finding balance in your exercise routine means finding a routine that works with your lifestyle. Everyone is going to miss a workout they had planned on doing and that's OK, life goes on. Once you find the right balance of days per week, minutes per day, and type of activity, you will wonder how others find exercising regularly so difficult. If you're concerned with "what is enough", consider the ACSM minimum recommendations of 150 minutes/week of low to moderate intensity or 20-60 minutes/week of high intensity exercise, or a combination of both (7). Remember the small things you can do to break up a long workday such as standing up and walking a bit every 30-45 minutes or including some light stretching every hour. Adding small amounts of activity to a day where you don't get to participate in structured exercise can add up to hundreds of extra burned calories over the course of a day. Those calories *will* add up.

Finding balance in your diet can be achieved by not depriving yourself of foods you enjoy eating for more than just a craving. This is why I encourage you to eat something you know isn't the best for your health a few times a week, give or take, depending on *you*, so you can stay sane while eating ~90% good, healthful, real food. Finding a balance means actually going out to eat with friends or family once in a while and not feeling bad about it (assuming you don't regularly go out to eat on your own). Finding a balance means eating food to fuel your body, make you feel good, and maintain a healthy weight without undue effort. Finding a balance also means finding what works for you and your family and how you can make eating healthy possible with different preferences and schedules.

Finding a balance with stress may be a bit more difficult, but I hope you've learned a few things to remind yourself of how simple (I didn't say easy) it is to handle a stressful situation. When you let someone get under your skin, whether they meant to or not, you lose every time. Your mood ends up ruined, not theirs. I still see people of all ages get stressed about things that once might have had an impact on me in some way, but now do not, and I believe it's never too late to change. It's not the circumstances, it's what you're made of.

Finding a balance with your outlook on life and day-to-day activities is a difficult thing to examine. The easiest way I can describe (different than the strategy itself) finding a balance in your outlook is to keep it in check. All it takes is seeing the silver lining and thinking about what you're thankful for and what you have to look forward to each day when you wake up and every night before you go to sleep. If you like to include this in your daily prayers, then by all means thank God for everything in your life; the food, the people you got to see that day, the health you've had during exercise, or safe driving. You can't control what happens to you, but you can control how you react to it.

Finding a balance with your motivation can be done by what I mentioned earlier; *accept* that you will have setbacks in all areas of life and *believe* that you will overcome those setbacks, learn from them, and be a better person than you used to be. Losing motivation doesn't doom you to fail because motivation can be regained. Giving up on a goal you have dooms you to fail at achieving that goal for the time being and it sets you further away than when you had started.

Finding balance with your lifestyle habits revolves around your daily schedule. If my examples of fitting in extra activity to break up a sedentary workday, finding a way to drink more water, or enjoying a hobby don't work for you, then brainstorm your own ideas and start applying them. The more you move, the better; and the less you move, the worse (to an extent, of course). Always remember, a positive habit that is done well 70% of the time, 7 days per week (you can always improve from there) is going to yield better results *over time* than a positive habit that is done perfectly 100% of the time on only 4 days of the week. You've heard it before, but it can't be stated enough: consistency is key.

The happiest people I know have learned how to balance their lives. They can manage time, relationships, and daily life with ease and without excessive stress. You can too; all it takes is a little practice and finding what works for *you*.

Denise was your classic example of an exercising couch potato. She exercised regularly and ate a typical "Western diet", which we all have heard has many flaws and unfortunately helps her maintain her overweight shape. Sure, she exercised by resistance training on weight machines for 30 minutes, twice per week and included 45 minutes of cardio 2-3 days per week as well, but that was a *very* small portion of her day – about 3-4% actually. Her diet wasn't perfect, like many of us, and she consistently ordered in food and drank soda and coffee drinks at work. The rest of the day outside of exercising she spent sitting at her desk, driving her car 15-20 minutes to work and back, sitting at the dinner table with her family, sitting down to "relax" and watch her favorite TV show after dinner, and sleeping.

Denise thinks she's doing herself a lot of good with her exercise schedule and doesn't understand why she doesn't see quick results. In a way, she is doing well. But in a whole other and cumulative way, she isn't. You see, when you exercise for 30-45 minutes per day, maybe 4-6 days per week, you find benefits. When you're sedentary the rest of your day and a large majority of your free time, it adds up and fights against what you earn in the gym, especially if you're eating a typical Western diet and just going through the motions when you exercise. She may burn 200-500 calories during those workouts, but what she's doing with the rest of her day is making the biggest difference in her long-term health.

If she were to stand up and stretch or walk around the office once every 45-60 minutes, find a somewhat active hobby to partake in, or even just stand and work at her desk she could easily burn an extra 100-200 calories a day, along with the added benefits of not developing a weak core, poor posture, lower back pain, rounded shoulders, tight chest muscles or tight hips that can all be a result of sitting too much. As you could imagine, not dealing with those issues would make a body feel a whole lot better when it actually does exercise. Not to mention, there is more and more research coming out that is showing the mental benefits of standing versus sitting (and/or taking standing breaks to break up periods of prolonged sitting). Who wouldn't want those added benefits of not sitting along with better mental focus at work?

I convinced Denise to first set an alarm on her phone and just try standing up and stretching out every hour. Once that was easy, I challenged her to walk around the office (which probably took 1-2 minutes) and then return to her desk once per hour. Soon enough, she didn't need an alarm and that extra movement became part of her day – and a part that she looked forward to. After only three weeks of taking my advice, she lost 25 pounds! See how easy it is?

Just kidding, that didn't happen. What did happen was a far more important step in the right direction. Denise noticed that she felt like pushing herself in the gym after work much more often than she used to. Her workout intensity picked up leading to more efficient and effective workouts. She felt more focused at her desk after moving every hour to break up the sitting. Most importantly, she improved one of her not-so-great lifestyle habits of sitting too much and noticed clear benefits after doing so. She then felt confident in her ability to improve her body composition, performance and lifestyle habits without the help of others. Now, how expensive are those treadmill desks?

Acknowledgements

First, I want to thank all of those who believe in my ability to share useful information regarding the subjects in this book. Without that support, it wouldn't have felt like a wise use of my time.

I want to thank all of the professors in the Kinesiology department at the University of Wisconsin - Eau Claire for the profound and life-changing experience you gave me and the outside-the-classroom learning opportunities you made so available to your students. You've encouraged your students to achieve excellence.

I'd like to thank everyone who is mentioned in the outlook section of this book. I never used to have the mindset I live with now, and it's greatly, in part, thanks to the situations and people I was surrounded with when "seeing the silver lining".

I want to thank everyone I've ever worked with up until this point in my life. The athletes, the personal training clients, the coaches and the teachers – I've learned something from all of you, whether you've realized it or not. You give me life and make continuously learning a meaningful endeavor.

Lastly, I want to thank my parents for their endless support thus far in everything I do inside and outside of my career. They've helped shape me into the person I am today and I couldn't be more grateful for the way I see the world around me.

Further reading on long-term physical maintenance:

Becoming a Supple Leopard, by Dr. Kelly Starrett with Glen Cordoza

http://www.mobilitywod.com/the-supple-leopard/

Deskbound, by Dr. Kelly Starrett with Juliet Starrett and Glen Cordoza

http://www.mobilitywod.com/deskbound/

Notes

Notes

References

Strategy 1: Exercise

1.   Zourdos, Michael C., et al. "Novel Resistance Training–Specific Rating of Perceived Exertion Scale Measuring Repetitions in Reserve." *The Journal of Strength & Conditioning Research* 30.1 (2016): 267-275.
2.   Shiraev, Tim, and Gabriella Barclay. "Evidence based exercise: Clinical benefits of high intensity interval training." *Australian Family Physician* 41.12 (2012): 960.
3.   Perry, Christopher GR, et al. "High-intensity aerobic interval training increases fat and carbohydrate metabolic capacities in human skeletal muscle." *Applied Physiology, Nutrition, and Metabolism* 33.6 (2008): 1112-1123.
4.   Giannaki, C. D., et al. "Eight weeks of a combination of high intensity interval training and conventional training reduce visceral adiposity and improve physical fitness: a group-based intervention." *The Journal of Sports Medicine and Physical Fitness* (2015).
5.   Woods, Jeffrey A., et al. "Cardiovascular exercise training extends influenza vaccine seroprotection in sedentary older adults: the immune function intervention trial." *Journal of the American Geriatrics Society* 57.12 (2009): 2183-2191.
6.   Nieman, David C., and Bente K. Pedersen. "Exercise and immune function." *Sports Medicine* 27.2 (1999): 73-80.
7.   Matthews CE, Ockene IS, Freedson PS, Rosal MC, Merriam PA, Hebert JR. "Moderate to vigorous physical activity and the risk of upper-respiratory tract infection." *Medicine & Science in Sports and Exercise* 34: 1242–1248, 2002.
8.   Kell, Robert T., Gordon Bell, and Art Quinney. "Musculoskeletal fitness, health outcomes and quality of life." *Sports Medicine* 31.12 (2001): 863-873.
9.   Ranganathan, Vinoth K., et al. "Effects of aging on hand function." *Journal of the American Geriatrics Society* 49.11 (2001): 1478-1484.
10. Stratton, John R., et al. "Cardiovascular responses to exercise. Effects of aging and exercise training in healthy men." *Circulation* 89.4 (1994): 1648-1655.
11. Ogawa, Takeshi, et al. "Effects of aging, sex, and physical training on car-

diovascular responses to exercise." *Circulation* 86.2 (1992): 494-503.

12. Stefanick, Marcia L., et al. "Effects of diet and exercise in men and post-menopausal women with low levels of HDL cholesterol and high levels of LDL cholesterol." *New England Journal of Medicine* 339.1 (1998): 12-20.

13. Thompson, PAUL D., et al. "The acute versus the chronic response to exercise." *Medicine and science in sports and exercise* 33.6 Suppl (2001): S438-45.

14. Radnor, John M., Rhodri S. Lloyd, and Jon L. Oliver. "Individual Response to Different Forms of Resistance Training in School-Aged Boys." *The Journal of Strength & Conditioning Research* 31.3 (2017): 787-797.

15. Lloyd, Rhodri S., et al. "Position statement on youth resistance training: the 2014 International Consensus." *British journal of sports medicine* (2013): bjsports-2013.

16. Lloyd, Rhodri S., et al. "Changes in sprint and jump performances after traditional, plyometric, and combined resistance training in male youth pre- and post-peak height velocity." *The Journal of Strength & Conditioning Research* 30.5 (2016): 1239-1247.

17. DiFiori, John P., et al. "Overuse injuries and burnout in youth sports: a position statement from the American Medical Society for Sports Medicine." *British journal of sports medicine* 48.4 (2014): 287-288.

18. LaPrade, Robert F., et al. "AOSSM early sport specialization consensus statement." *Orthopaedic journal of sports medicine* 4.4 (2016): 2325967116644241.

19. **Connolly, Declan AJ, Stephen E. Sayers, and Malachy P. McHugh. "Treatment and prevention of delayed onset muscle soreness." *The Journal of Strength & Conditioning Research* 17.1 (2003): 197-208.**

20. Miernik, Marta, et al. "Massage therapy in myofascial TMD pain management." *Advances in clinical and experimental medicine: official organ Wroclaw Medical University* 21.5 (2011): 681-685.

21. MacDonald, Graham Z., et al. "An acute bout of self-myofascial release increases range of motion without a subsequent decrease in muscle activation or force." *The Journal of Strength & Conditioning Research* 27.3 (2013): 812-821.

22. MacDonald, Graham Z., et al. "Foam rolling as a recovery tool after an intense bout of physical activity." *Med Sci Sports Exerc* 46.1 (2014): 131-142.

23. Pearcey, Gregory EP, et al. "Foam rolling for delayed-onset muscle soreness and recovery of dynamic performance measures." *Journal of athletic training* 50.1 (2015): 5-13.

24. Healey, Kellie C., et al. "The effects of myofascial release with foam rolling

on performance." *The Journal of Strength & Conditioning Research* 28.1 (2014): 61-68.

25. "Essentials of Strength Training and Conditioning." *National Strength and Conditioning Association.* Third edition. 2008.

Strategy 2: Diet

1. Miura, J., et al. "The long-term effectiveness of combined therapy by behavior modification and very low-calorie diet: 2 years follow-up." *International Journal of Obesity* 13.Suppl 2 (1989): 73-77.

2. Johns, David J., et al. "Diet or exercise interventions vs combined behavioral weight management programs: a systematic review and meta-analysis of direct comparisons." *Journal of the Academy of Nutrition and Dietetics* 114.10 (2014): 1557-1568.

3. Slavin, J. L. "Position of the American Dietetic Association: health implications of dietary fiber." *Journal of the American Dietetic Association* 108.10 (2008): 1716-1731.

4. Arnaud, M. J. "Mild dehydration: a risk factor of constipation?" *European Journal of Clinical Nutrition* 57 (2003): S88-S95.

5. Woo, Hye-Im, et al. "A Controlled, Randomized, Double-blind Trial to Evaluate the Effect of Vegetables and Whole Grain Powder That Is Rich in Dietary Fibers on Bowel Functions and Defecation in Constipated Young Adults." *Journal of cancer prevention* 20.1 (2015): 64.

6. Chandalia, Manisha, et al. "Beneficial effects of high dietary fiber intake in patients with type 2 diabetes mellitus." *New England Journal of Medicine* 342.19 (2000): 1392-1398.

7. Cordain, Loren, et al. "Origins and evolution of the Western diet: health implications for the 21st century." *The American Journal of Clinical Nutrition* 81.2 (2005): 341-354.

8. Centers for Disease Control and Prevention (CDC). "National diabetes fact sheet: national estimates and general information on diabetes and prediabetes in the United States, 2011." *Atlanta, GA: US Department of Health and Human Services, Centers for Disease Control and Prevention* 201 (2011).

9. **Centers for Disease Control and Prevention.** *National Diabetes Statistics Report: Estimates of Diabetes and Its Burden in the United States, 2014.* **Atlanta, GA: U.S. Department of Health and Human Services; 2014.**

10. American Diabetes Association. "2. Classification and diagnosis of diabetes." *Diabetes Care* 39. Supplement 1 (2016): S13-S22.

11. Espeland, Mark A., et al. "Impact of an intensive lifestyle intervention on use and cost of medical services among overweight and obese adults with type 2 diabetes: the action for health in diabetes." *Diabetes Care* 37.9 (2014): 2548-2556.

12. Berardi, John, and Ryan Andrews. "The Essentials of Sport and Exercise Nutrition." *Toronto: Precision Nutrition* (2010).

13. DellaValle, Diane M., Liane S. Roe, and Barbara J. Rolls. "Does the consumption of caloric and non-caloric beverages with a meal affect energy intake?" *Appetite* 44.2 (2005): 187-193.

14. Dennis EA, Dengo AL, Comber DL, et al. Water consumption increases weight loss during a hypocaloric diet intervention in middle-aged and older adults. *Obesity (Silver Spring)*. 2010;18:300–307.

15. Davy BM, Dennis EA, Dengo AL, et al. Water consumption reduces energy intake at a breakfast meal in obese older adults. *J Am Diet Assoc.* 2008;108:1236–1239.

16. Armstrong, Lawrence E. "Challenges of linking chronic dehydration and fluid consumption to health outcomes." *Nutrition reviews* 70.suppl 2 (2012): S121-S127.

17. Duncan, Glen E., et al. "Exercise training, without weight loss, increases insulin sensitivity and postheparin plasma lipase activity in previously sedentary adults." *Diabetes Care* 26.3 (2003): 557-562.

18. Aragon, Alan Albert, and Brad Jon Schoenfeld. "Nutrient timing revisited: is there a post-exercise anabolic window." *Journal of the International Society of Sports Nutrition* 10.1 (2013): 5.

19. Katz, David L., et al. "Effects of egg ingestion on endothelial function in adults with coronary artery disease: A randomized, controlled, crossover trial." *American heart journal* 169.1 (2015): 162-169.

20. Berger, Samantha, et al. "Dietary cholesterol and cardiovascular disease: a systematic review and meta-analysis." *The American journal of clinical nutrition* (2015): ajcn100305.

21. Barber, Fedricker Diane. "Effects of social support on physical activity, self-efficacy, and quality of life in adult cancer survivors and their caregivers." *Oncology Nursing Forum.* Vol. 40. No. 5. 2013.

22. Anderson, Eileen S., et al. "Social-cognitive determinants of physical activity: the influence of social support, self-efficacy, outcome expectations, and self-regulation among participants in a church-based health promotion study." *Health Psychology* 25.4 (2006): 510.

23. Springer, Andrew E., Steven H. Kelder, and Deanna M. Hoelscher. "Social support, physical activity and sedentary behavior among 6th-grade girls: a

cross-sectional study." *International Journal of Behavioral Nutrition and Physical Activity* 3.1 (2006): 8.

24. Héroux, M., et al. "A personalized, multi-platform nutrition, exercise, and lifestyle coaching program: A pilot in women." *Internet Interventions* 7 (2017): 16-22.

Strategy 3: Stress

1. Björntorp, Per. "Metabolic implications of body fat distribution." *Diabetes Care* 14.12 (1991): 1132-1143.
2. Epel, Elissa S., et al. "Stress and body shape: stress-induced cortisol secretion is consistently greater among women with central fat." *Psychosomatic medicine* 62.5 (2000): 623-632.
3. Lupien, Sonia J., et al. "The effects of stress and stress hormones on human cognition: Implications for the field of brain and cognition." *Brain and cognition* 65.3 (2007): 209-237.
4. Falconier, Mariana K., et al. "Stress from daily hassles in couples: Its effects on intradyadic stress, relationship satisfaction, and physical and psychological well being." *Journal of marital and family therapy* 41.2 (2015): 221-235.
5. Herbert, Tracy Bennett, and Sheldon Cohen. "Stress and immunity in humans: a meta-analytic review." *Psychosomatic Medicine* 55.4 (1993): 364-379.
6. Torres, Susan J., and Caryl A. Nowson. "Relationship between stress, eating behavior, and obesity." *Nutrition* 23.11 (2007): 887-894.
7. Dallman, Mary F. "Stress-induced obesity and the emotional nervous system." *Trends in Endocrinology & Metabolism* 21.3 (2010): 159-165.
8. Wardle J, Gibson EL. "Impact of stress on diet: processes and implications." In: Stansfeld SA, Marmot M (eds). *Stress and the Heart*. BMJ Books: London, 2002, pp. 124–149.

Strategy 6: Lifestyle Habits

1. Ellenbogen, Jeffrey M. "Cognitive benefits of sleep and their loss due to sleep deprivation." *Neurology* 64.7 (2005): E25-E27.
2. Lo, June C., John A. Groeger, Nayantara Santhi, Emma L. Arbon, Alpar S. Lazar, Sibah Hasan, Malcolm Von Schantz, Simon N. Archer, and Derk-Jan Dijk. "Effects of partial and acute total sleep deprivation on performance across cognitive domains, individuals and circadian phase." *PloS one* 7.9 (2012): e45987.

3.   Dunstan, David W., Alicia A. Thorp, and Genevieve N. Healy. "Prolonged sitting: is it a distinct coronary heart disease risk factor?." *Current opinion in cardiology* 26.5 (2011): 412-419.

4.   Duvivier, Bernard M. F. M., Nicolaas C. Schaper, Michelle A. Bremers, Glenn Van Crombrugge, Paul P. C. A. Menheere, Marleen Kars, and Hans H. C. M. Savelberg. "Minimal intensity physical activity (standing and walking) of longer duration improves insulin action and plasma lipids more than shorter periods of moderate to vigorous exercise (cycling) in sedentary subjects when energy expenditure is comparable." *PloS one* 8.2 (2013): e55542.

5.   Bailey, Daniel P., David R. Broom, Bryna C.r. Chrismas, Lee Taylor, Edward Flynn, and John Hough. "Breaking up prolonged sitting time with walking does not affect appetite or gut hormone concentrations but does induce an energy deficit and suppresses postprandial glycaemia in sedentary adults." *Applied Physiology, Nutrition, and Metabolism* ja (2015).

6.   Arnaud, M. J. "Mild dehydration: a risk factor of constipation?" *European Journal of Clinical Nutrition* 57 (2003): S88-S95.

7.   http://www.acsm.org/about-acsm/media-room/news-releases/2011/08/01/acsm-issues-new-recommendations-on-quantity-and-quality-of-exercise